Integrated Intraoperative Ocular Coherence Tomography for Pediatric Ocular Surgery

Developments in Ophthalmology

Vol. 61

Series Editor

F. Bandello Milan

Integrated Intraoperative Ocular Coherence Tomography for Pediatric Ocular Surgery

Volume Editor

Ken K. Nischal Pittsburgh, PA

36 figures, 36 in color, 2021

Karger

Basel · Freiburg · Hartford · Oxford · Bangkok · Dubai · Kuala Lumpur · Melbourne · Mexico City · Moscow · New Delhi · Paris · Shanghai · Tokyo

Ken K. Nischal
UPMC Children's Hospital of Pittsburgh
Children's Hospital Drive
45th & Penn Avenue
CHP Faculty Pavilion, Suite 5000
Pittsburgh, PA 15201 (USA)

Disclosure Statement

This book project is sponsored in part by Carl Zeiss AG

Library of Congress Cataloging-in-Publication Data

Names: Nischal, Ken K., editor.
Title: Integrated intraoperative ocular coherence tomography for pediatric ocular surgery / volume editor, Ken K. Nischal.
Other titles: Developments in ophthalmology ; v. 61. 0250-3751
Description: Basel ; Hartford : Karger, 2021. | Series: Developments in ophthalmology, 0250-3751 ; vol. 61 | Includes bibliographical references and indexes. | Summary: "This book is about the use of i2OCT (i.e., integrated intraoperative optical coherent tomography) for pediatric ophthalmic surgery. Such surgery demands precision and a greater degree of certainty to ensure that it has a positive and long-lasting outcome for the child. The use and incorporation of i2OCT presents an opportunity to achieve a better result. While the subspecialties of retina and cornea have been targeted as fields within ophthalmology that would clearly benefit from i2OCT, this technology can be used in almost every subspecialty of ophthalmology. This book has chapters about the use of i2OCT for strabismus surgery, for oculoplastic surgery, and miscellaneous uses that can be applied for ocular surface issues in pediatric cataract and for the evaluation of glaucoma drainage devices"-- Provided by publisher.
Identifiers: LCCN 2021003910 (print) | LCCN 2021003911 (ebook) | ISBN 9783318068535 (hardcover ; alk. paper) | ISBN 9783318068542 (ebook)
Subjects: MESH: Tomography, Optical Coherence--methods | Ophthalmologic Surgical Procedures | Child
Classification: LCC R857.O6 (print) | LCC R857.O6 (ebook) | NLM W1 DE998NG v.61 2021 | DDC 616.07/545--dc23
LC record available at https://lccn.loc.gov/2021003910
LC ebook record available at https://lccn.loc.gov/2021003911

Bibliographic Indices. This publication is listed in bibliographic services, including Current Contents® and MEDLINE/Pubmed.

www.karger.com
Printed on acid-free and non-aging paper (ISO 9706)
ISSN 0250–3751
e-ISSN 1662–2790
ISBN 978–3–318–06853–5
e-ISBN 978–3–318–06854–2

Contents

Published online: February 15, 2021

Integrated Intraoperative Ocular Coherence Tomography for Pediatric Ocular Surgery. Dev Ophthalmol. Basel, Karger, 2021, vol 61, pp VI–VIII (DOI: 10.1159/000511814)

Introduction

The advent of a portable optical coherent tomography (OCT) brought with it a new access and ability to image the eye in the operating room. The problem with the devices that were available to do this was that the surgeon had to move the microscope away in order to perform the imaging of the eye by one or more devices. This created a bottleneck and disruption to the normal surgical flow. The step that we as surgeons had been waiting for was the ability to integrate OCT technology so that simultaneous viewing of the surgical field and the OCT image could be performed. This would allow for a better understanding of the anatomy of the eye that was being operated on, and also allow a safer environment in which to perform surgery. The term intraoperative OCT does not do justice to the fact that this technology is now integrated into the microscope, and so the terms integrated intraoperative OCT, or i^2OCT, or microscope-integrated OCT, or MI-OCT, are being used to differentiate it from other forms of intraoperative OCT, namely the handheld varieties that are available. Commercially available spectral-domain i^2OCT/MI-OCT systems include the Haag-Streit iOCT (Haag-Streit, Koeniz, Switzerland), Leica EnFocus (Leica Microsystems, Buffalo Grove, IL, USA), and Zeiss RESCAN 700 (Carl Zeiss Meditec, Jena, Germany).

I am delighted to write an introduction to a book dedicated to the use of i^2OCT for pediatric ophthalmic surgery. Pediatric ophthalmic surgery demands precision and a greater degree of certainty to ensure that the surgery that is being conducted has a positive and long-lasting outcome for the child.

Whereas it is long accepted that there is a learning curve for all trainees and all junior attendings (and even senior attendings when they attempt more complex surgery), the use and incorporation of i^2OCT flattens this learning curve and therefore – especially in pediatric ocular surgery – presents an opportunity to achieve a better result than one might have without i^2OCT.

There are those who would argue that without some sort of controlled trial one could not say definitively that the use of i^2OCT does indeed improve outcomes in children. However, the DISCOVER study [1] clearly demonstrates improved outcomes in adults. Similarly, the chapters in this book demonstrate very clearly that there is a level of understanding and a demonstration of techniques which per say give the surgeon a degree of security that is not available without this technology.

While the subspecialties of retina and cornea have been targeted as fields within ophthalmology that would clearly benefit from i^2OCT, the interesting and perhaps most exciting thing about this technology is that it can be used in almost every subspecialty of ophthalmology. In this book there are chapters about the use of i^2OCT for strabismus surgery, for oculoplastic surgery, and a chapter about the miscellaneous uses that can be applied for ocular surface issues in pediatric cataract and also for the evaluation of glaucoma drainage devices.

It is important to understand that there are two ways to use any technology that is integrated into the operating microscope. One way is to view the image on a screen whereby the surgeon moves his or her head away from the oculars to be able to see the OCT image. However, I feel a more sophisticated and a much better utilization of the technology is to view the integrated OCT images while looking down the oculars and viewing the surgical field at the same time. The understanding and acknowledgement that ocular dominance plays a role in determining how comfortably a surgeon can do this is extremely important. Most of us who are right handed are right eye dominant and the image that is displayed in the commercially available microscopes is indeed in the right ocular. This can lead to a degree of confusion and it is probably the reason why many surgeons prefer to look up than to look through the oculars. While the ideal solution would be that any system that has i^2OCT would include the ability to switch the display from one ocular to the other depending on the ocular dominance of the surgeon, one can play an optical trick by adding +1 or +2 to the refractive power of the oculars; the surgeon looks at the surgical field without the OCT image and focusses on the surgical field adding either +1D or +2D to the ocular power (the older surgeon will be able to cope with the +1 and the younger surgeon with the +2). When the surgeon now adds the OCT image, and relaxes a little to look at the subsequent image, it results in an optical separation of the two images. This can make it more comfortable to use the oculars simultaneously to look at the surgical field and the OCT image.

The next issue is the display color of the OCT image. It has long been known in the visual display unit industry that red-green displays fatigue our visual system and that a better option would be the grayscale. While either display can be used, it is interesting that many older surgeons prefer the red-green to the grayscale. As long as one is aware of the fatigue that red-green displays can cause the user, I do not think it matters which is used since both adequately show good images.

The last point of discussion is whether there needs to be special surgical instruments created to allow surgery while the OCT is being used so as to reduce the amount of light scatter. Remember OCT is a light-based technology and of course one would expect that metal or titanium instruments cause a shadow effect. You will see in some of the chapters and the examples given that this is not necessarily true, and that surgery can be conducted while viewing the OCT image in cases where the cornea (for example) is opaque or has scarring in it.

In essence, the advantages of i^2OCT are that they allow a young trainee or young attending to have a flatter learning curve as they operate on children's eyes, and therefore give children the best opportunity not to be adversely affected by somebody's learning curve. The other advantage for established surgeons is that it allows the completion and even the attempt at more complex surgeries that perhaps the surgeon would have been reluctant to attempt or even not contemplated at all, having explained to the parents and the patient that the risk of something going wrong was too high for the surgeon to attempt the surgery. Again, there are examples throughout the following chapters where surgery was performed when perhaps without the use of i^2OCT it would have been practically impossible to have done so.

While the use of i^2OCT will increase in the next 5–10 years, the advancement of the technology to a heads-up display where the OCT image can be rendered not only in 2D but also in 3D will bring this technology even more quickly into mainstream practice on a daily basis.

Ken K. Nischal, MD, FAAP, FRCOphth

UPMC Children's Hospital of Pittsburgh, PA, USA

Reference

1 Ehlers JP, Modi YS, Pecen PE, et al: The DISCOVER Study 3-year results: feasibility and usefulness of microscope-integrated intraoperative OCT during ophthalmic surgery. Ophthalmology 2018; 125:1014–1027.

Published online: February 23, 2021

Integrated Intraoperative Ocular Coherence Tomography for Pediatric Ocular Surgery. Dev Ophthalmol. Basel, Karger, 2021, vol 61, pp 1–7 (DOI: 10.1159/000511821)

Integrated Intraoperative Optical Coherence Tomography for Pediatric Lamellar Corneal Transplant Surgery

Gerald W. Zaidman

Department of Ophthalmology, Westchester Medical Center, New York Medical College, Valhalla, NY, USA

Abstract

Integrated intraoperative anterior segment optical coherence tomography is an extremely valuable tool that can be used by corneal surgeons when performing pediatric lamellar corneal transplant surgery. This chapter will demonstrate its use in infants and children with a variety of corneal diseases. These diseases include congenital corneal opacities such as Peters' anomaly (both types I and II), surgical management of limbal dermoids, and its use in selective corneal transplant surgery such as DALK (deep anterior lamellar keratoplasty) or DSEK (Descemet stripping endothelial keratoplasty). These techniques could be used in children with anterior corneal scarring or storage disorders, such as mucopolysaccharidoses, or posterior endothelial disease, such as congenital hereditary endothelial dystrophy or posterior polymorphous dystrophy. This chapter will demonstrate the author's experience using this device during anterior segment corneal surgery.

Optical coherence tomography (OCT) was introduced in 1991 to assist in imaging the posterior segment of the eye. Anterior segment OCT (AS-OCT) became available about 10 years ago. AS-OCT enabled non-contact and indirect visualization and evaluation of structures within the anterior segment, from the cornea to the anterior portion of the lens [1]. Initially, there were two types of AS-OCTs available. Both were imaging systems designed to be used in the office, though one type could be attached or incorporated into a slit-lamp rather than be used as an independent device. Its initial use was primarily in identifying anomalies of the iris and the anterior chamber. However, with the development of selective corneal transplant surgery such as DSAEK (Descemet stripping automated endothelial keratoplasty), DMEK (Descemet membrane endothelial keratoplasty), and DALK (deep anterior lamellar keratoplasty), the device was modified so that it could be attached to the operating microscope and used with those surgical procedures. In 2018, the ophthalmic literature evaluated and reported on various models of microscope-integrated OCT systems [2]. Zeiss incorporated an OCT system into their ReScan microscope. The integrated OCT ReScan system is helpful in all forms of corneal transplant surgery. Reports have described its use on patients with Fuchs' dystrophy, bullous keratopathy, keratoconus, DSAEK, and DMEK [3]. Although these are diseases primarily of adults, we have demonstrated the successful use of the ReScan system on corneal transplant surgery in infants and children. Here I will discuss our experience with this technology.

Scenarios

Although it can be used in the office during the preoperative evaluation of the patient, the primary value of AS-OCT technology is its use in the operating room during corneal transplant surgery. It is a safe, non-invasive technology, incorporated into the operating microscope, which allows the corneal surgeon to image the layers of the cornea during the surgical procedure. In essence, it serves a role similar to that served by the slit-lamp in imaging the layers of the cornea in the office. This technology improves the diagnosis and the surgical decision-making process in adults and now, more recently, children. It decreases the surgical time and surgical complication rate in the operating room in children undergoing these procedures and increases the success rate. I will present my experience using intraoperative AS-OCT in children with corneal disorders.

The three main indications for corneal transplant surgery in children are congenital corneal opacities (CCO), acquired non-traumatic corneal opacities, and acquired traumatic corneal opacities. Adults with similar disorders can be evaluated in the office by a slit-lamp examination, ultrasonography, ultrasound biomicroscopy, or office-based OCT when we are planning for surgery. In an adult with a dense corneal scar, a slit-lamp examination is possible. This enables you to determine if there is scarring or synechiae from the iris to the angle or if there are iridocorneal adhesions. Additionally, the slit-lamp examination will help you determine if a cataract is present and if there is any synechiae from the iris to the lens. However, this is often not possible in children. They can be extremely uncooperative and difficult to examine, especially younger children. Therefore, surgical decision making in a child is usually based on an exam under anesthesia typically using all of the necessary diagnostic devices. The results of the exam under anesthesia are then brought into the operating room. Surgery then commences with the concurrent use of integrated AS-OCT. This modality allows the surgeon to image the corneal and anterior segment pathology, helping direct surgical techniques and improving the surgical outcome.

In my experience, two-thirds of the children with CCO have a form of anterior segment dysgenesis such as Peters' anomaly or sclerocornea. Another large group is children with dermoids. One-sixth of the children with CCO will have corneal endothelial disorders such as congenital hereditary endothelial dystrophy (CHED) or posterior polymorphous dystrophy (PPMD). Finally, there is a small group of children with corneal opacification secondary to herpes, trauma, or storage disorders such as mucopolysaccharidosis or macular dystrophy.

In the management of children with congenital opacities, the surgeon is often unable to recognize corneal adhesions or congenital cataracts. This makes the intraoperative AS-OCT extraordinarily important. The intraoperative AS-OCT helps the surgeon visualize these structures and helps the surgeon plan for the patient's surgery – it makes the surgery more predictable and successful. I routinely use the OCT after I enter the anterior chamber and after I have injected viscoelastic into the anterior chamber. I then take a spatula and pass it between the cornea and the iris to break any synechiae that are present in the

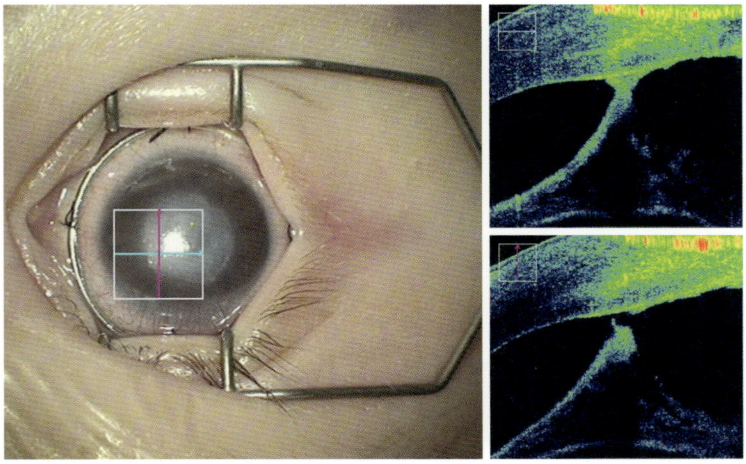

Fig. 1. A child with CCO due to iridocorneal adhesions seen very easily on OCT.

child's eye (Fig. 1). This makes the subsequent steps of the anterior segment surgery much safer and improves the success rate.

Additionally, in those patients with type 2 Peters anomaly, in which there are lenticular adhesions to the cornea, the intraoperative OCT is extraordinarily valuable. While one is doing the anterior segment dissection, one can use the OCT to help visualize the adhesions of the lens to the cornea and visualize where the lens is positioned in the vitreous cavity. This will enable intraoperative dissection to proceed more carefully and safely as one performs the case.

The first case is a patient with a CCO due to an anterior segment dysgenesis (Fig. 1). In this case of Peters anomaly type I there is no lenticular involvement, but there are iridocorneal adhesions. As one can see in these images, the preoperative ultrasound biomicroscopy demonstrated synechiae from the iris to the cornea and no evidence of a cataract. The AS-OCT demonstrated the same findings. By localizing the position of the synechiae, the surgeon was able to appropriately cut those before removing the patient's scarred cornea and replacing it with a corneal graft. In contrast, sometimes in a case of a CCO the AS-OCT may not demonstrate any iridocorneal adhesions and no lenticular involvement. The imaging reassures the surgeon that it is unlikely that during the keratoplasty there will be a need for iris surgery or lenticular surgery. Therefore, this makes the surgical planning more straightforward.

Infants or children with corneal scars can have very unusual anterior segments. If the preoperative exam demonstrates involvement of anterior chamber structures or the lens, intraoperative AS-OCT can help the surgeon localize the exact position of the anterior segment pathology and direct the surgeon's approach on how to best excise the surgical scar and complete the corneal transplant.

Congenital limbal dermoids are not a rare occurrence in infants and children. In some parts of the world they are the major reason for anterior segment and corneal surgery in infants and children. As we know, a dermoid is a choristoma in which a variety of soft tissue structures have migrated to the periphery of the cornea, usually the inferotemporal quadrant, and this choristoma is then "stuck" onto the cornea, typically involving only the anterior corneal layers. Once again, the difficulty of evaluating these infants and small children in the office is ever present. It is very helpful to have an intraoperative AS-OCT available at the time of surgery. In this way, one can get

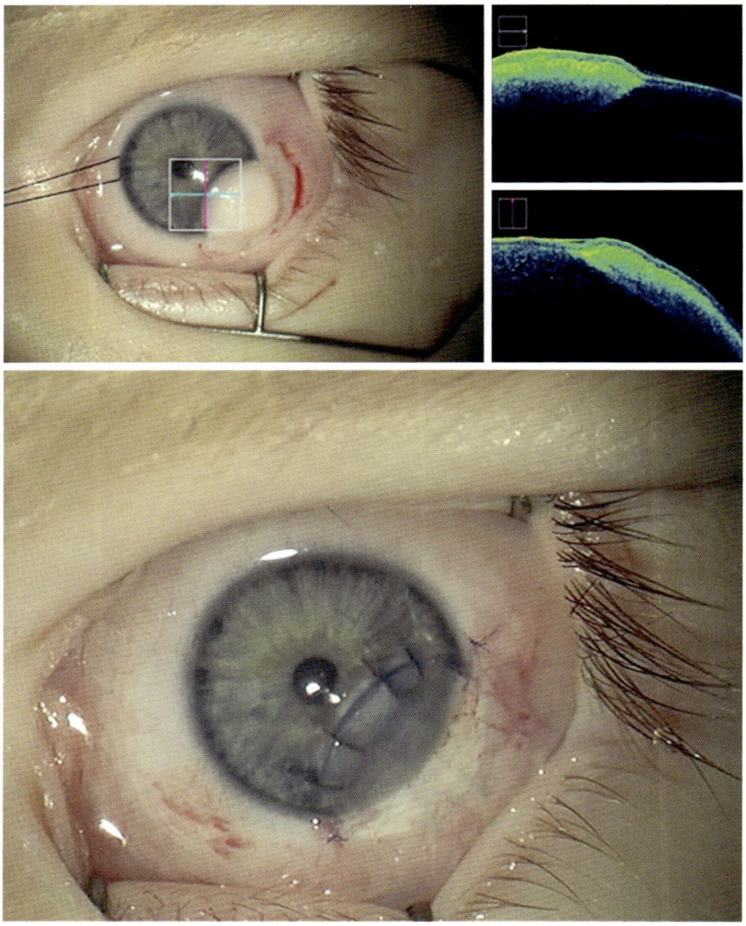

Fig. 2. This shows the dermoid on the corneal surface and its corresponding OCT. The OCT shows the depth of the dermoid into the peripheral cornea and sclera, and demonstrates that the dermoid has not penetrated through the cornea. This allows the surgeon to finish the case with a lamellar keratoplasty.

an impression of how deep the dermoid penetrates into the sclera and whether or not it penetrates through the cornea into the anterior chamber or into the sclera. In my experience, most congenital limbal dermoids do not penetrate into the anterior chamber of the eye, but they usually penetrate to about two-thirds or three-quarters of the depth of the patient's peripheral cornea and sclera. As demonstrated in this patient (Fig. 2), the intraoperative AS-OCT shows that the dermoid has not gone past the posterior cornea. Therefore, a lamellar keratectomy with a lamellar corneal transplant can be used to remove the dermoid without entering the anterior chamber and give a good cosmetic result. The intraoperative AS-OCT demonstrates how deep the dermoid goes into both the peripheral cornea and the sclera.

Another use for the intraoperative integrated AS-OCT is when planning a selective corneal transplant in children. Selective corneal transplants are generally performed in two groups of patients, most of whom are adults – anterior lamellar scarring, including keratoconus, and endothelial disorders. DALK is used in patients with anterior corneal disorders, most frequently keratoconus. It can also be used in anterior corneal scarring, or opacification of the cornea from various metabolic or storage disorders, such as mucopolysaccharidosis, Hurler's syndrome (Fig. 3),

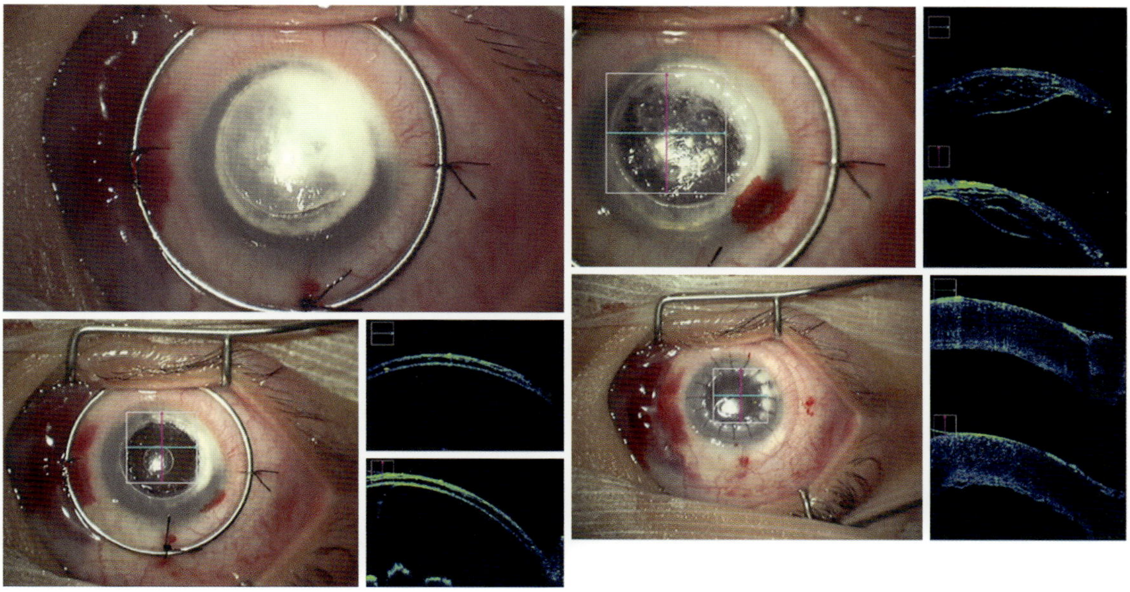

Fig. 3. This shows a child with Sly syndrome, mucopolysaccharidosis type VII. The composite demonstrates the surgical steps during DALK using a big bubble technique, with OCT imaging. It shows the air injection followed by creation of the big bubble. We can then see residual Descemet membrane and endothelium after excision of the corneal stroma. The final photo shows the end of the case after the donor cornea has been sutured into position.

or macular corneal dystrophy. If one can accomplish a lamellar keratoplasty (such as a DALK), one can eliminate the risks of endothelial graft rejection and traumatic wound rupture for the child's life. The other group of selective corneal transplants is patients with corneal edema due to endothelial decompensation. In adults this would be Fuchs' corneal dystrophy, and in children either CHED or PPMD.

Figure 3 shows a child with mucopolysaccharidosis type VII, otherwise known as Sly syndrome, in whom a DALK was performed. The surgery starts by imaging the patient's cornea with AS-OCT and determining the approximate depth of the deposits. A big bubble technique is then used to isolate the anterior corneal layers and excise them leaving just Descemet membrane and endothelium behind, as can be seen in these photos, and then doing a lamellar keratoplasty. This procedure has the benefits of decreasing corneal rejection rates since the endothelium is not transplanted. This technique can also be used in children with keratoconus who do not have deep corneal scarring.

The last group of children who may be candidates for a selective transplant will be those with endothelial disorders such as CHED or PPMD. In contrast to adults who have endothelial keratoplasty, children who undergo endothelial grafts cannot be expected to lie flat on their backs for any period of time. It is usually quite difficult to do a slit-lamp exam on these children on the first postoperative day to determine the position of the endothelial graft. Therefore, the AS-OCT imaging increases the surgeon's ability to determine the position of the endothelial graft. As a result, I routinely use the intraoperative AS-OCT in any child who is having an endothelial graft for CHED or PPMD. The photos shown in Figure 4 are an adult patient with Fuchs dystrophy who is phakic

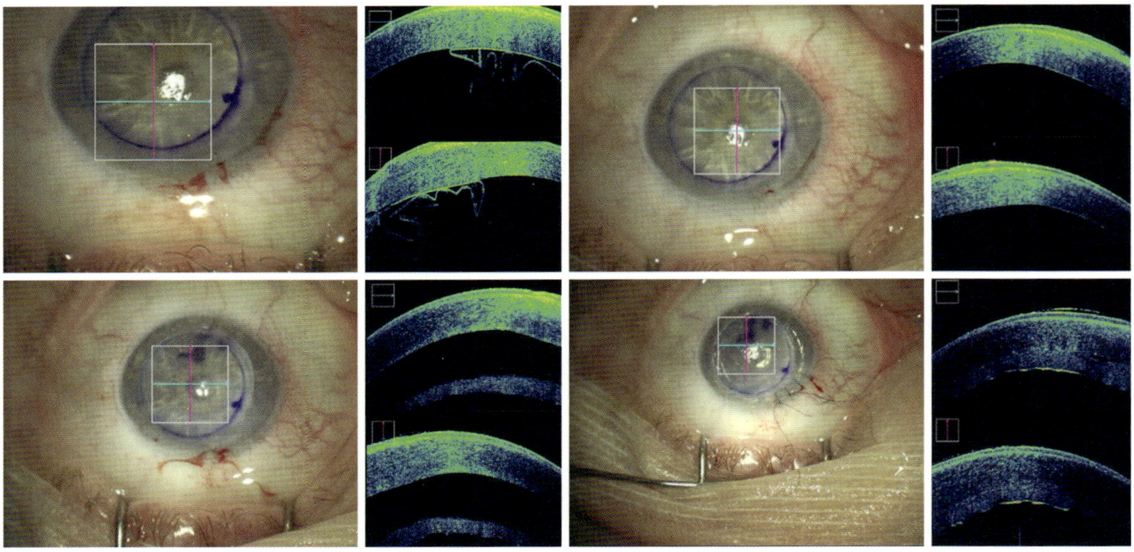

Fig. 4. This demonstrates an endothelial keratoplasty on an adult with Fuchs' dystrophy. The OCT imaging shows removal of Descemet membrane (top left), then the bare stroma (top right). Insertion of the donor cornea into the anterior segment (bottom left), and the final position of the donor cornea attached to the recipient corneal stroma with an air bubble in the anterior chamber (bottom right).

since that would be most analogous to a child with PPMD or CHED. One can see that the integrated AS-OCT demonstrates Descemet membrane as it has been partially removed from the cornea. It helps us determine if the surgeon has successfully removed the Descemet membrane and the endothelium. The donor cornea is then taken and placed in position, and you can see the endothelial donor graft lying in the anterior chamber. After inflating the anterior chamber with a large bubble of air, the corneal endothelium has now been successfully opposed to the corneal stroma. I have used the integrated AS-OCT in a similar fashion in children with PPMD or CHED.

In closing, the use of intraoperative AS-OCT has been extremely helpful in the management of infants and children with corneal disorders. It has shortened the surgical time and increased the surgical success rate leading to decreased surgical complications and better patient results. In my experience, its use can facilitate both novice and experienced surgeons in achieving excellent surgical outcomes and decreasing the learning curve.

Conflict of Interest Statement

The author has no financial disclosure pertaining to this work.

Author Contributions

G.W.Z. fulfilled the following: (1) substantial contributions to the conception or design of the work; or the acquisition, analysis, or interpretation of data for the work; (2) drafting the work or revising it critically for important intellectual content; (3) final approval of the version to be published.

References

1 Doors M, Berendschot TTJM, de Brabander J, et al: Value of optical coherence tomography for anterior segment surgery. J Cataract Refract Surg 2010;36:1213–1229.

2 Ehlers JP, Modi YS, Pecen PE, et al: The DISCOVER study 3-year results: feasibility and usefulness of microscope-integrated intraoperative OCT during ophthalmic surgery. Ophthalmology 2018;125:1014–1027.

3 Patel AS, Goshe JM, Srivastava JM, Ehlers JP: Intraoperative optical coherence tomography-assisted Descemet membrane endothelial keratoplasty in the DISCOVER study: first 100 cases. Am J Ophthalmol 2020;210:167–173.

Gerald W. Zaidman
Westchester Ophthalmology
40 Saw Mill River Road
Hawthorne, NY 10532 (USA)
pedkera@aol.com

Published online: February 16, 2021

Integrated Intraoperative Ocular Coherence Tomography for Pediatric Ocular Surgery. Dev Ophthalmol. Basel, Karger, 2021, vol 61, pp 8–14 (DOI: 10.1159/000511817)

Current Knowledge about the Anterior Interface in Children Operated for Congenital Cataract

Marie-José Tassignon Luc Van Os

Department of Ophthalmology of the Antwerp University Hospital, University of Antwerp, Antwerp, Belgium

Abstract

The relationship between the anterior vitreous interface and the posterior capsule has received increasing attention in the past decade. The advent of integrated intraoperative optical coherence tomography has allowed a real-time opportunity to grasp this dynamic understanding. Here we describe the normal anatomy of this interface in children and then demonstrate the variation in this interface with different forms of pediatric cataract, namely a posterior plaque and posterior capsular opacity due to abnormal adherence to the vitreous face. The authors describe these changes using meticulous annotation. An understanding of these differences will aid the surgeon in managing pediatric cataracts in a more confident and safe manner.

Children born with cataract need special care because they are at risk of developing poor vision if their cataract is not operated in time. Congenital cataract is a rare disease and can be related to a lot of known gene defects. The compendium of human genes, called the Online Mendelian Inheritance in Man (OMIM), is a very handy source of information on inherited congenital cataracts. OMIM is a comprehensive, authoritative compendium of human genetic phenotypes that is freely available and updated daily. OMIM is authored and edited at the McKusick-Nathans Institute of Genetic Medicine, Johns Hopkins University School of Medicine, under the direction of Dr. Ada Hamosh, and its official home is at omim.org.

The drawback of this compendium is that it only collects published or proven human genetic phenotypes. However, not all types of congenital cataract have been associated with genetic anomalies. As an example, the pathology we will discuss in more length in this chapter, the "anterior, vitreolenticular, interface dysgenesis" (AVLID) has not yet been associated with any specific human gene defect and is most probably caused by errors in the multiplication of somatic cells involved in the development of the anterior interface. The cause for this error in cell multiplication remains unknown.

Another issue is terminology – there is currently no universally accepted international classification for pediatric cataract, which complicates comparison between different studies and outcomes. In 2016, Lin et al. [1] proposed a novel congenital cataract classification based on the phenotype of the cataract and more specifically on the location of the lens opacities. We are very much in favor of this classification because it is straightforward and easy to use. However, each classification has its shortcomings. For example, this classification does not consider anomalies of the anterior interface, which is related to specific aspects of congenital cataracts with plaque formation.

It should be mentioned that the anterior interface has only been studied very recently. Observations of this interface were primarily related to the use of the bag-in-the-lens (BIL) technology, which was first developed in adults. All details and history of BIL can be find in the book published in 2019 by Springer in their series "Innovative Implantation Techniques" and edited by both authors of this chapter [2].

Our first experience of BIL in children was published in 2007 [3]. Because of the excellent results obtained in this small cohort of patients, we continued to use the BIL in pediatric cataract cases and learned more about its benefits, indication, and complications over the years.

With the advent of intraoperative optical coherence tomography (OCT), it was possible to observe the presence of the anterior interface. In 2011, Dick and Schultz [4] described this interface when using the femtosecond laser to operate some forms of congenital cataracts. The OCT images observed in femtosecond laser devices are monodirectional frozen images while the OCT images observed preoperatively with the Lumera Zeiss (Zeiss, Germany) microscope are bidirectional video recordings out of which images can be frozen. It was first described in adults in 2016 by Tassignon and Ní Dhubhghaill [5].

There is a consensus amongst pediatric cataract surgeons that performing a primary posterior continuous circular capsulorhexis (PPCCC) is a must in pediatric cataract [6]. However, the anatomy behind the posterior capsule remains a black box for most surgeons. It was Wieger [7] who wrote his PhD thesis in 1883 on the ligament attaching the anterior hyaloid and the posterior capsule in adults. In 1887, Berger [8] then described the retrolenticular space (Fig. 1) defined by the posterior capsule and the anterior hyaloid. This space was later defined as the Berger space.

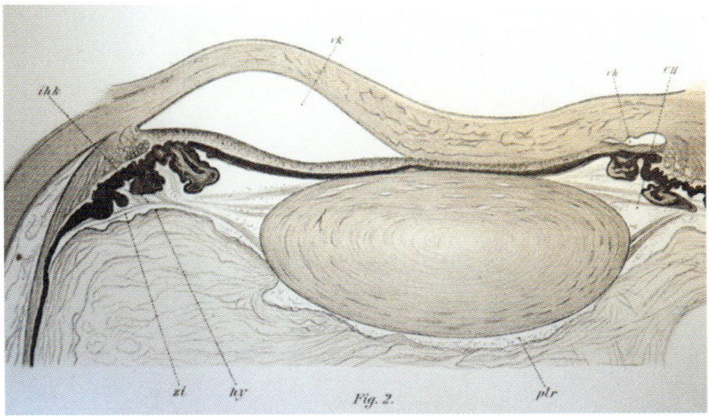

Fig. 1. The Berger space [8, p. 29–30].

The long-term results of the BIL in pediatric cataract were published in 2016 with exceptionally good results, such as very few cases of secondary cataract and good visual outcomes even in unilateral cataracts [9]. The same authors focused on eyes presenting with posterior plaque types of cataract as described by Morrison [10] in 2011. After careful dissection of the posterior capsule including the plaque, they applied immunohistochemical analysis on these plaques and found vitreous collagen embedded in them. They concluded that these plaques can be considered a repair mechanism of both vitreous and lens to close existing defects of the posterior capsule and/or anterior hyaloid [11]. When applying proteomics analysis on these plaques they found that this repair mechanism was caused by mesenchymal cells originating either form the lens (lens epithelial cells) or from the vitreous (histiocytes) [12].

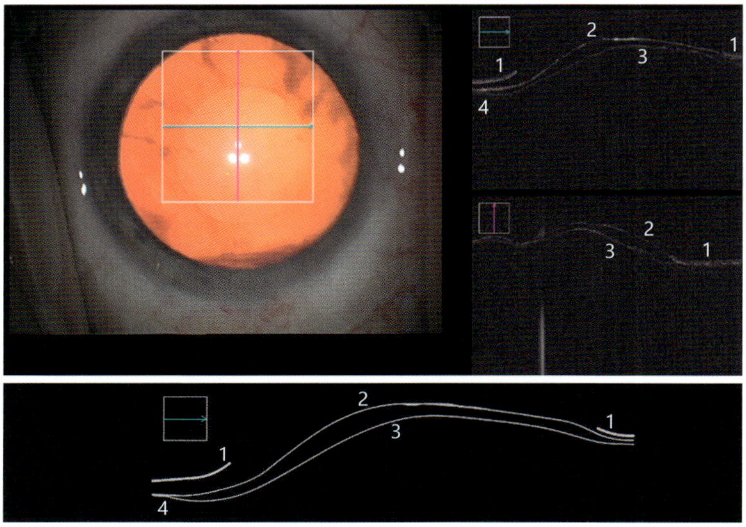

Fig. 2. OCT image of a juvenile cataract anterior interface: 1, anterior capsule after performing anterior capasulorhexis; 2, posterior capsule prior to performing PPCCC; 3, anterior hyaloid; 4, attachment of posterior capsule and anterior hyaloid, also called the Wieger attachment.

We were thus able to clarify the so far unexplained subtle signs of anterior vitreous face disturbance during posterior capsulorhexis in pediatric cataract surgery, as described in 2008 by Praveen et al. [13]. When looking at the surgical video recordings of pediatric cases operated by the same group, they were able to define the incidence of vitreolenticular interface dysgenesis in their cohort of pediatric cases performed in a tertiary setting [14]. This incidence was as high as 52.9%, out of which 72.4% were found in unilateral cataract cases and in 90% of children with posterior plaques.

Clinical Cases

Case 1: Normal Anatomy

In normal young children the anatomy of the anterior interface is comparable to the adult, but the size of the Berger space is often much smaller. Figure 2 shows an OCT capture (Zeiss Lumera, Germany) of an eye operated from a juvenile cataract. We can easily recognize the anterior capsule (1), the posterior capsule (2), and the anterior hyaloid membrane (3). In addition, this image beautifully shows the Wieger attachment (4) between the posterior capsule and anterior hyaloid.

When pushing back the anterior hyaloid from the posterior capsule with an ophthalmic viscosurgical device (OVD; Healon Regular, Bausch & Lomb, USA), after puncturing the posterior capsule and injecting the OVD through this small capsule hole, the anterior hyaloid is visibly separated from the posterior capsule (Fig. 3). This maneuver allows a safe PPCCC without having to fear damaging the anterior hyaloid.

These images clearly illustrate the value of intraoperative OCT in distinguishing the different anatomical landmarks of the vitreolenticular interface. In cases with a normal interface, this mostly serves as an illustration and is not essential for performing surgery. In more complex cases where the vitreolenticular interface is abnormal, the OCT can provide valuable help to achieve successful surgery.

Case 2: Posterior Plaque

Figure 4 shows an OCT image taken after the lens material has been removed from the capsular bag, leaving only the posterior plaque and the posterior capsule. The plaque can be seen at the lens side as well as at the vitreous side of the posterior capsule. This image shows the repair mechanism closing the gap in the posterior cap-

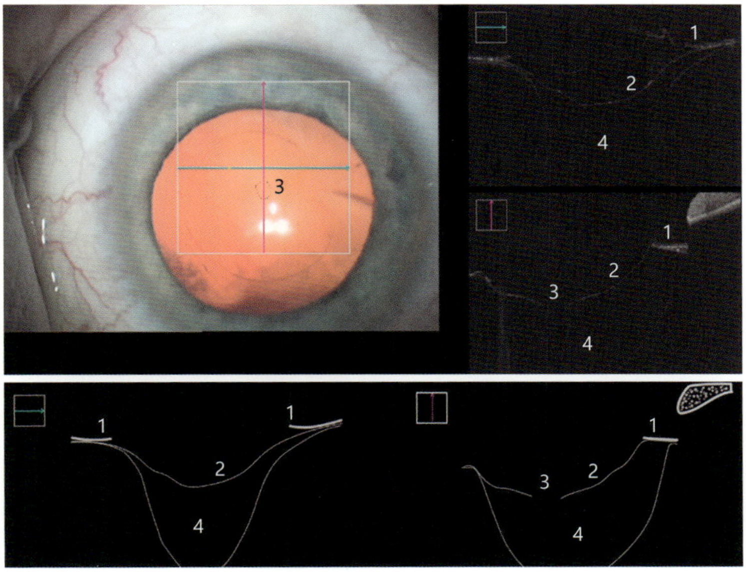

Fig. 3. Anterior hyaloid separated from the posterior capsule: 1, anterior capsule after having performed an ACCC; 2, posterior capsule; 3, posterior capsule hole; 4, space between posterior capsule and anterior hyaloid.

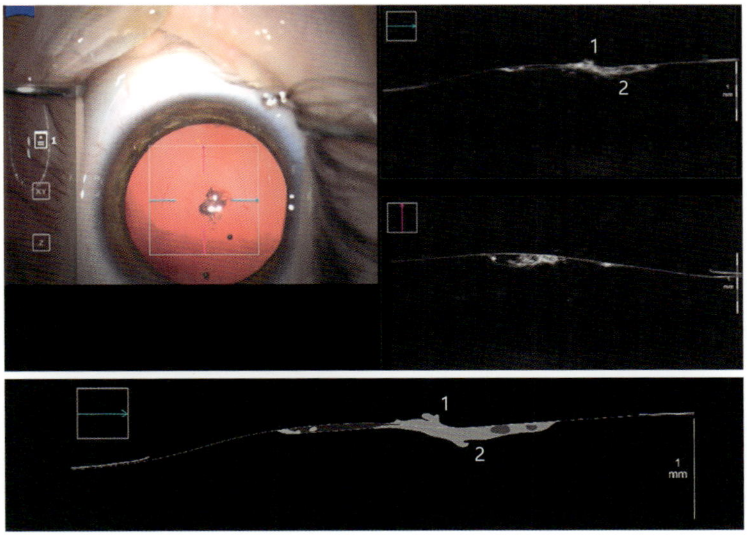

Fig. 4. Typical case of anterior interface dysgenesis. Posterior plaque is present above (1) and under (2) the posterior capsule on OCT.

sule (1) and the anterior hyaloid (2). This is a typical case of anterior interface dysgenesis in a posterior capsule plaque type of congenital cataract.

When finding the cleavage plane between the posterior capsule and the anterior hyaloid in the previous case, we were surprised to discover another opening at the level of the anterior hyaloid (Fig. 5). This opening allowed us to inflate another space, called the Erggelet space. This space corresponds to the connection between the Cloquet canal and the anterior hyaloid [15].

Case 3: Abnormal Adherence between the Posterior Capsule and Anterior Hyaloid

Figure 6 shows the eye of a 2-year-old child after removal of the lens material. The posterior capsule is pulled downwards almost in a triangular

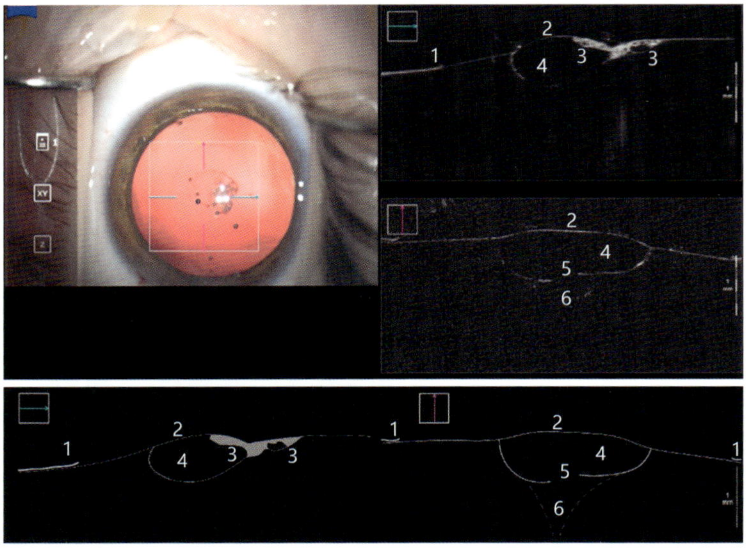

Fig. 5. Opening at the level of the anterior hyaloid: 1, anterior capsule; 2, posterior capsule; 3, plaque lining at the posterior face of the posterior capsule; 4, inflated space with OVD between the posterior capsule and anterior hyaloid; 5, hole in the anterior hyaloid; 6, Erggelet space corresponding to the chalice of the Cloquet canal ending at the anterior hyaloid.

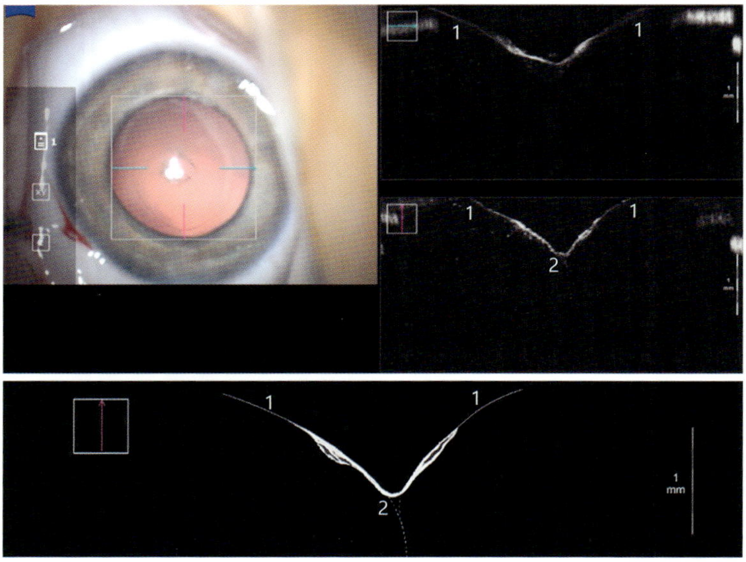

Fig. 6. Eye of a 2-year-old child after removal of the lens material: 1, posterior capsule; 2, thin strand dragging the posterior capsule downwards, corresponding to remnants of the Erggelet space/Cloquet canal.

shape. A small line can be distinguished behind the posterior capsule. This corresponds to the Erggelet space/Cloquet canal, with remnants of poorly resolved tertiary vitreous.

After puncturing the posterior capsule, OVD was injected behind the posterior capsule, which could then be partly separated from the anterior hyaloid. This is illustrated in Figure 7. Note that the anterior hyaloid appears to be very thick on this image.

Complete separation of the posterior capsule and anterior hyaloid could not be obtained; however, a PPCCC could be performed, leaving an intact but very thick anterior hyaloid (Fig. 8). The edge of the posterior rhexis can be distinguished in the photograph (green dashed line), but not on the OCT. This is most likely because they were strongly adherent. To enable proper positioning of the BIL implant, an anterior vitrectomy was

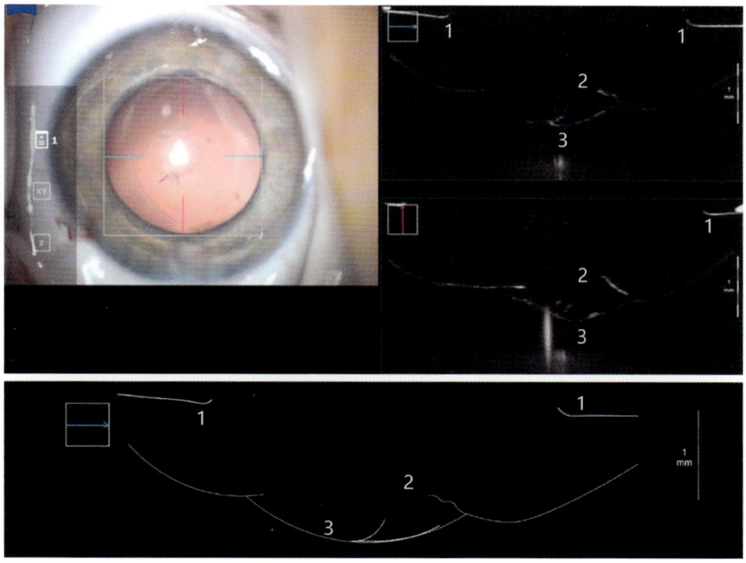

Fig. 7. The posterior capsule partly separated from the anterior hyaloid: 1, edge of the anterior capsulorhexis; 2, puncture of the posterior capsule; 3, anterior hyaloid.

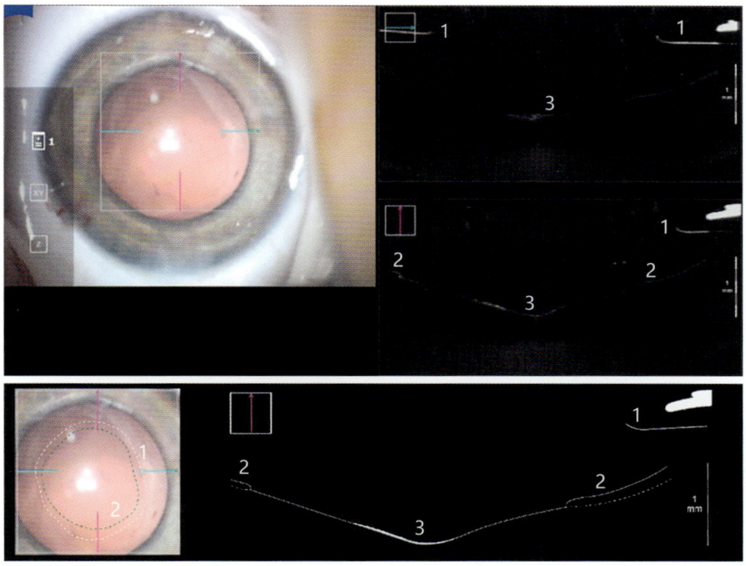

Fig. 8. PPCCC: 1, edge of the anterior capsulorhexis (white dashed line in lower photograph); 2, edge of the posterior capsulorhexis (green dashed line); 3, thick anterior hyaloid.

performed consisting of the removal of the adherent anterior hyaloid to the posterior capsule. This resulted in relaxation of the posterior capsule. Thereafter, a BIL could be implanted as expected.

Conclusion

Integrated intraoperative OCT during pediatric cataract surgery reveals new insights about the variations in the anatomy of the vitreoretinal interface. It also allows us to understand normal and abnormal development of the anterior interface corresponding to the development of the different stages of vitreous development. This provides valuable information that will help in performing safe and successful surgery.

Acknowledgements

The authors would like to thank ophthalmologist Dr. Diana Carmen Dragnea for helping in providing the technical drawings for the figures.

Conflict of Interest Statement

Intellectual property for bag-in-the-lens and ring calipers is licensed to Morcher, Germany. A consultancy agreement exists with Théa and Ziemer.

Author Contributions

M.-J.T. and L.V.O. fulfilled all of the following: (1) substantial contributions to the conception or design of the work; or the acquisition, analysis, or interpretation of data for the work; (2) drafting the work or revising it critically for important intellectual content; (3) final approval of the version to be published.

References

1 Lin H, Duoru L, Liu Z, Long E, et al: A novel congenital cataract category system based on lens opacity locations and relevant anterior segment characteristics. Invest Ophthalmol Vis Sci 2016;57:6389–6395.
2 Tassignon M-J, Ní Dhubhghaill S, Van Os L: Innovative Implantation Technique: Bag-in-the-Lens Cataract Surgery. Berlin, Springer, 2019.
3 Tassignon MJ, De Veuster I, Godts D, Kosec D, Van den Dooren K, Gobin L: Bag-in-the-lens intraocular lens implantation in the pediatric eye. J Cataract Refract Surg 2007;33:611–617.
4 Dick HB, Schultz T: Primary posterior laser-assisted capsulotomy. J Refract Surg 2014;30:128–134.
5 Tassignon MJ, Ní Dhubhghaill S: Real-time intraoperative optical coherence tomography imaging confirms older concepts about the Berger space. Ophthalmic Res 2016;56:222–226.
6 Vasavada AR, Praveen MR, Tassignon M-J, et al: Posterior capsule management in congenital cataract surgery. J Cataract Refract Surg 2011;37:173–193.
7 Wieger G: Über den Canalis Petiti und ein “Ligamentum hyaloideocapsulare,” thesis, Kaiser Wilhelm University, Strasbourg, 1883.
8 Berger E: Beiträge zur Anatomie des Auges in Normalem und Pathologischem Zustande. Wiesbaden, Bergmann, 1887.
9 Van Looveren J, Ní Dhubhghaill S, Godts D, et al: Pediatric bag-in-the-lens intraocular lens implantation: long-term follow-up. J Cataract Refract Surg 2015; 41:1685–1692.
10 Morrison DG, Lambert SR, Wilson ME: Posterior capsular plaque in bilateral congenital cataracts. J AAPOS 2012;16:17–20.
11 Van Looveren J, Van Gerwen V, Timmermans JP, Tassignon MJ: Immunohistochemical characteristics of the vitreolenticular interface in congenital unilateral posterior cataract. J Cataract Refract Surg 2016;42:1037–1045.
12 Van Looveren J, Van Gerwen V, Schildermans K, Laukens K, Baggerman G, Tassignon MJ: Proteomic analysis of posterior capsular plaques in congenital unilateral cataract. Acta Ophthalmol 2018;96:e963–e969.
13 Praveen MR, Vasavada AR, Koul A, Trivedi RH, Vasavada VA, Vasavada VA: Subtle signs of anterior vitreous face disturbance during posterior capsulorhexis in pediatric cataract surgery. J Cataract Refract Surg 2008;34:163–167.
14 Van Looveren J, Vael A, Ideler N, Sillen H, Mathysen D, Tassignon MJ: Influence of the vitreolenticular interface in pediatric cataract surgery. J Cataract Refract Surg 2018;44:1203–1210.
15 Erggelet H: Befunde bei fokaler Beleuchtung mit der Gullstrandschen Nernstspaltlampe. Klin Monatschr Augenheilk 1914;53:II.

Marie-Jose Tassignon
Antwerp University and University Hospital of Antwerp
Wilrijkstraat 10
BE–2650 Edegem, Antwerp (Belgium)
marie-jose.tassignon@uza.be

Published online: March 1, 2021

Integrated Intraoperative Ocular Coherence Tomography for Pediatric Ocular Surgery. Dev Ophthalmol. Basel, Karger, 2021, vol 61, pp 15–25 (DOI: 10.1159/000511818)

Pediatric Vitreoretinal Surgery and Integrated Intraoperative Optical Coherence Tomography

Sophie Cai[a] Anthony Therattil[a, b] Lejla Vajzovic[a]

[a]Retina Division, Duke Eye Center, Durham, NC, USA; [b]New York Medical College School of Medicine, Valhalla, NY, USA

Abstract

Intraoperative portable handheld and microscope-integrated OCT enhance the pediatric vitreoretinal surgeon's diagnostic abilities during examination under anesthesia and surgery, particularly in children who are challenging to examine preoperatively due to young age or ocular trauma. Improved OCT-guided visualization of vitreoretinal anatomic relationships has the potential to improve surgical safety and efficiency. In retinopathy of prematurity and other pediatric retinal vascular conditions, intraoperative OCT can be critical for distinguishing between retinoschisis and retinal detachment and highlighting abnormalities of the vitreoretinal interface that may contribute to development of tractional retinal detachments. During retinal detachment repair, intraoperative OCT aids identification of subtle retinal breaks, residual subretinal fluid, retained perfluorocarbon, preretinal membranes, and residual hyaloid, among other findings. In macular surgery, intraoperative OCT has demonstrated value in confirming completion or lack thereof of epiretinal and internal limiting membrane peeling and differentiating between lamellar and full-thickness macular holes. OCT-guided subretinal bleb formation and genetic vector delivery are critical to ensuring accurate localization of subretinal gene delivery for inherited retinal degenerations. Research on development of OCT-compatible surgical instruments, real-time three-dimensional volumetric OCT imaging, and integration with intraoperative OCT angiography are anticipated to further increase the utility of intraoperative OCT in pediatric vitreoretinal surgical decision-making.

Optical coherence tomography (OCT) has revolutionized the clinical and surgical diagnosis and management of retinal disease, with growing applications in the field of pediatric retina in particular. In the operating room, the introduction of the portable handheld OCT, such as the commercially available spectral-domain Bioptigen/Leica Envisu c2300 (Bioptigen Inc., Research Trial Park, NC, USA; Fig. 1a), has greatly improved

Sophie Cai and Anthony Therattil contributed equally to this work.

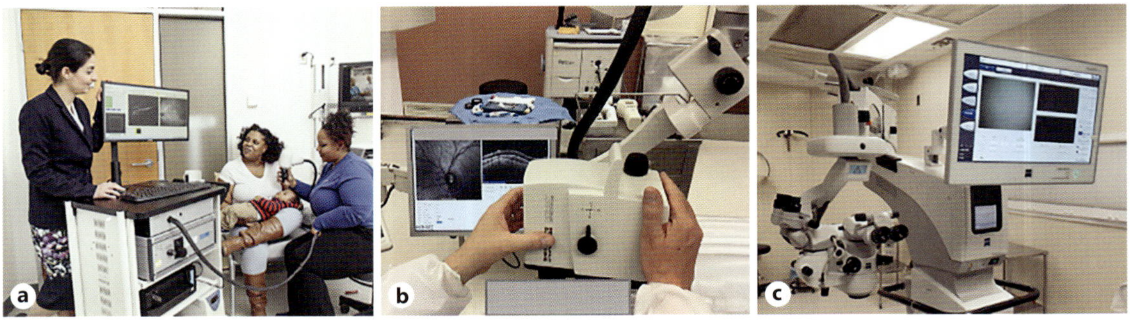

Fig. 1. Intraoperative OCT modalities. Representative spectral-domain OCT devices suitable for imaging pediatric patients in the operating room include: the commercially available portable handheld Bioptigen/Leica Envisu c2300 (**a**), investigational portable Heidelberg Spectralis Flex module (**b**), and commercially available MIOCT Zeiss RESCAN 700 system, coupled with the Zeiss OPMI LUMERA 700 surgical microscope (**c**).

the resolution with which retinal pathology can be characterized during examinations under anesthesia [1, 2]. With the addition of a sterile cover or specialized mount attaching the portable OCT probe to a surgical microscope, high-resolution handheld OCT images can be acquired during pauses in vitreoretinal surgery [3]. The investigational Heidelberg Spectralis Flex module (Heidelberg Engineering, Heidelberg, Germany; Fig. 1b), a portable armature-based device, features a flexible arm that permits multi-directional spectral-domain OCT imaging, integrated with standardized retinal thickness map analysis as well as multimodal angiographic imaging if desired. Several research groups have also developed handheld swept-source OCT and OCT angiography probes that are faster, higher resolution, and lighter and more ergonomically comfortable for the imager than the commercially available spectral-domain Bioptigen/Leica Envisu c2300 device [4].

Shared challenges of the aforementioned portable handheld OCT systems are the need to pause surgery to perform OCT imaging and the inability to directly overlay OCT images onto the surgical field as visualized through the microscope oculars. By contrast, microscope-integrated OCT (MIOCT) permits the real-time projection of horizontal and vertical OCT B-scans from an area of interest through the microscope oculars, allowing simultaneous viewing with the surgical field [5]. Commercially available spectral-domain MIOCT systems include the Haag-Streit iOCT (Haag-Streit, Koeniz, Switzerland) [6], Leica EnFocus (Leica Microsystems, Buffalo Grove, IL, USA) [7], and Zeiss RESCAN 700 (Carl Zeiss Meditec, Jena, Germany; Fig. 1c) [8]. In currently available MIOCT systems, the surgeon uses the foot pedal to control lateral localization of the desired region of interest of OCT imaging, but focusing in the axial direction may require a second assistant [9]. Investigational high-speed swept-source MIOCT systems have also been developed and tested for both static widefield [10] and real-time non-widefield imaging [5, 11, 12].

Advances in MIOCT technology and the potential for coupling with heads-up displays on high-definition external monitors (Ngenuity, Alcon, Fort Worth, TX, USA) [13] are ushering in an exciting era for what researchers at the Duke Eye Center have called 4D-MIOCT, or volumetric real-time OCT imaging, to improve vitreoretinal surgical precision, safety, and efficiency [14, 15]. Pediatric vitreoretinal surgery particularly stands to benefit from 4D-MIOCT given the unique technical challenges, such as a firmly adherent posterior hyaloid and the practical difficulties of obtaining comprehensive imaging in the clinic pre- and postoperatively to guide surgical management and postoperative monitoring. Here, we review diagnostic and therapeutic applications of MIOCT in pediatric vitreoretinal surgery, as well as highlight areas in need of further research.

Diagnostic and Therapeutic Uses of Intraoperative OCT

Among children for whom young age, lack of cooperation, and/or recent ocular trauma may preclude detailed retinal examination in the clinic, intraoperative portable handheld OCT during examination under anesthesia can be critical for the diagnosis and quantitative characterization of pediatric retinal pathology requiring surgical or procedural management (Fig. 2). In addition to confirming or ruling out surgical conditions such as retinal detachments, epiretinal membranes (Fig. 2a), full-thickness macular holes, and submacular or subhyaloid hemorrhages (Fig. 2b), OCT is helpful for diagnosing pediatric choroidal neovascular membranes with associated leakage that may require intravitreal anti-vascular endothelial growth factor (VEGF) injections under sedation [16, 17]. The growing use of OCT to image children with retinal vascular diseases such as retinopathy of prematurity (ROP) has also highlighted the power of OCT to help identify and monitor neovascularization, which can inform decision-making regarding the need for laser photocoagulation or intravitreal anti-VEGF treatment [18, 19].

Surgically, intraoperative OCT has a broad range of diagnostic and therapeutic applications to pediatric retina. In children with ROP, OCT is transforming our ability to detect subtle vitreoretinal pathology that may not be detectable by indirect ophthalmoscopy [20–22]. A recent study revealed that a subset of infants diagnosed with

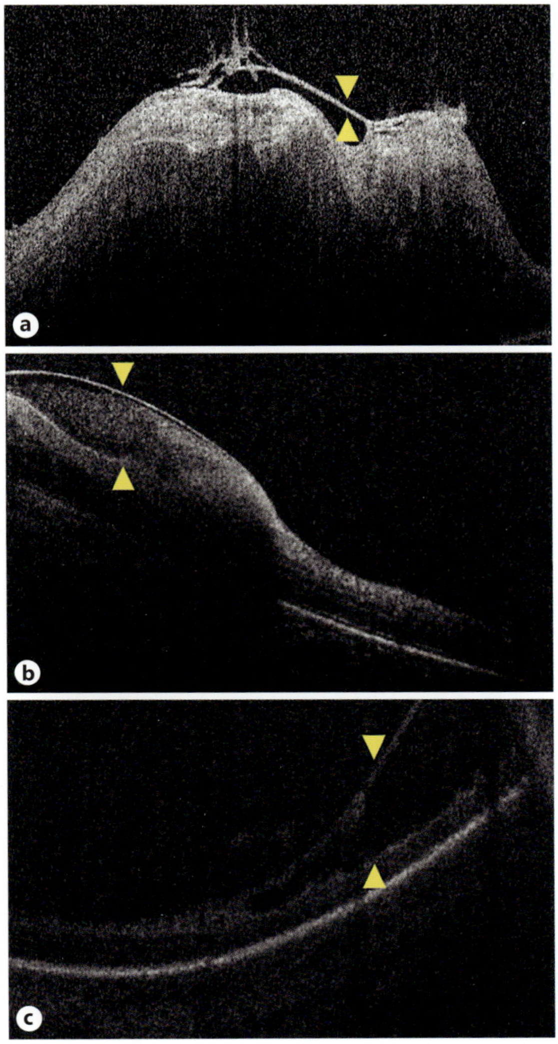

Fig. 2. Portable OCT imaging of pediatric patients. **a** An intraoperative OCT image taken with the Heidelberg Spectralis Flex module demonstrates an epiretinal membrane (arrowheads) in the setting of combined hamartoma of retina and retinal pigment epithelium in an 8-year-old child who subsequently underwent pars plana vitrectomy with epiretinal membrane peeling. Handheld Bioptigen/Leica Envisu c2300 OCT images demonstrate subhyaloid hemorrhage (arrowheads) secondary to non-accidental trauma in a 10-month-old child (**b**) and peripheral retinoschisis (arrowheads) without retinal detachment in a 3-month-old ex-24-weeker with history of ROP (**c**).

stage 4 ROP by traditional indirect ophthalmoscopy in fact had retinoschisis, rather than retinal detachment, based on handheld OCT imaging (Fig. 2c) [23]. Further research is needed to clarify the prognosis and optimal management of eyes with ROP-associated retinoschisis without retinal detachment. Among patients with ROP-associated retinal detachment, OCT has also been shown to provide more definitive assessment than indirect ophthalmoscopy of whether the fovea is involved, thus enabling the distinction between stage 4A and 4B ROP [23]. Ultra-widefield handheld OCT prototypes [24] can enhance the visualization of peripheral tractional preretinal membranes and vitreous abnormalities that may contribute to the pathology of ROP-associated retinal detachments, and thus inform the approach of pediatric vitreoretinal surgeons to vitrectomy and membrane peeling [20, 21, 25, 26].

Intraoperative OCT also holds promise for detailed visualization of the vitreoretinal interface in complex tractional retinal detachments associated with hereditary pediatric retinal vascular diseases such as familial exudative vitreoretinopathy (FEVR). OCT of patients with FEVR has been previously shown to be useful in diagnosing vitreoschisis, vitreoretinal and vitreopapillary traction, and shallow retinal detachments that can be challenging to diagnose by fundus examination [27, 28]. Intraoperative OCT guidance may improve the safety and efficiency of vitrectomy in patients with FEVR-associated retinal detachments by helping surgeons to localize safe planes of membrane dissection and areas of particularly strong vitreoretinal adhesion.

Analogous advantages apply to incorporation of intraoperative OCT during vitrectomies for serous retinal detachments associated with congenital optic disc anomalies. In a case report of MIOCT-assisted surgical repair of a serous retinal detachment in the setting of morning glory syndrome, MIOCT was used to guide careful trimming of the vitreous in areas of strong vitreopapillary and vitreoretinal adhesion [29]. Intraoperative OCT was also noted to provide helpful feedback to the surgeon during delicate epiretinal membrane peeling over areas of retinoschisis. In serous retinal detachments associated with optic disc pit maculopathy, when drainage of relatively shallow subretinal fluid is required, intraoperative OCT can aid localization of the highest point of subretinal fluid before selecting a drainage retinotomy site. OCT guidance is also valuable for assessing whether the subretinal fluid has been adequately drained [30].

In rhegmatogenous retinal detachments associated with certain underlying pediatric inherited retinal diseases, intraoperative OCT can be essential for identifying subtle causative retinal breaks. A published series of macular hole-associated retinal detachments in children under the age of 5 years with Knobloch syndrome reported a case where an oblique slit full-thickness macular hole was visible only on OCT and not by clinical examination [31]. In advanced stages of choroideremia, extensive loss of fundus pigmentation can make macular holes or small retinal breaks associated with retinal detachments challenging to visualize without OCT [32]. Similarly, previous literature has highlighted the difficulty of finding retinal breaks preoperatively and intraoperatively in retinal detachments associated with ocular and oculocutaneous albinism [33], a process that could benefit from the use of OCT to scan the area of retinal detachment. In retinal detachments associated with chorioretinal colobomas, where retinal breaks often arise from the intercalary membrane within the coloboma [34, 35] but have also been reported elsewhere [36], intraoperative OCT can aid the identification of small breaks difficult to visualize against the background of the coloboma.

In addition to facilitating the localization of retinal breaks, intraoperative OCT can increase the safety and precision of multiple other steps of retinal detachment repair. The DISCOVER (Determination of Feasibility of Intraoperative Spectral Domain Microscope Combined/Integrated OCT Visualization during en face Retinal and Ophthalmic Surgery) study of adult retinal detachment repairs reported the utility of intraoperative OCT for aiding the confirmation of posterior vitreous detachment, identification of preretinal membranes, identification of the need for retinectomy, confirmation of retinal reattachment or identification of persistent subretinal fluid, and distinction between subretinal fluid and intraretinal edema or retinoschisis [37–39]. Intraoperative OCT has been used to identify retained perfluorocarbon bubbles [40] as well as provide real-time guidance during the surgical removal of loculated perfluorocarbon bubbles [41]. During surgical repair of diabetic tractional retinal detachments, MIOCT can help identify safe planes of dissection and vitreoschisis [42] and provide real-time feedback on the extent of tissue deformation during membrane peeling [43]. MIOCT-assisted determination of whether iatrogenic full-thickness breaks have been created during membrane peeling can also influence decision-making about the need for gas tamponade [43].

For macular hole repair, the DISCOVER study reported that intraoperative OCT findings altered the surgical management of 12% of adult cases by either confirming the completion of membrane peel or revealing residual membranes when the surgeon was uncertain of whether further peeling was required [37]. Surgeons additionally reported intraoperative OCT to be useful in visualizing the vitreoretinal interface, confirming the release of vitreomacular traction, measuring the size of the macular hole after membrane peeling, and identifying the location of the internal limiting flap when internal limiting membrane peeling was performed. In a case report detailing the surgical management of a pediatric traumatic macular hole, the surgeon used intraoperative handheld OCT to find that the macular hole was nearly closed at the conclusion of surgery, resulting in the decision to end the case with fluid-air exchange without longer-acting gas tamponade [44]. At the postoperative 1-month follow-up visit, the macular hole was noted to be successfully closed. Although further research is needed to assess the correlation between intraoperative macular hole closure and long-term visual acuity and anatomic outcomes, the potential for using intraoperative OCT findings to guide the need for gas tamponade after macular hole repair in children may help alleviate the challenges of pediatric postoperative patient positioning and decrease chance of cataract formation.

Similar to macular hole repair, the PIONEER (Prospective Intraoperative and Perioperative Ophthalmic Imaging and Optical Coherence Tomography) study showed that microscope-mounted portable OCT imaging provided valuable intraoperative feedback during epiretinal membrane peeling in adult patients [45]. Intraoperative OCT in this study was shown to reveal residual membranes needing peeling in 12% of cases and to show the absence of residual membrane in 9% of cases, avoiding unnecessary surgical manipulation [45]. Pediatric epiretinal membranes (Fig. 2a), for which pars plana vitrectomy with membrane peel can yield favorable visual acuity outcomes [46, 47], are notably more challenging to peel than adult epiretinal membranes [48, 49]. Not only is the posterior hyaloid typically attached in children, but it is also thicker and more adherent to underlying retina and retinal vessels than in adults with epiretinal membranes [47, 49–53]. Intraoperative MIOCT can aid the confirmation of full posterior vitreous detachment induction and also facilitate visualization of the epiretinal membrane anatomy with respect to the underlying retina, permitting more confident dissection (Fig. 3).

In the setting of pediatric ocular trauma or non-accidental trauma, intraoperative OCT can contribute to the diagnosis and management of traumatic macular holes, epiretinal membranes,

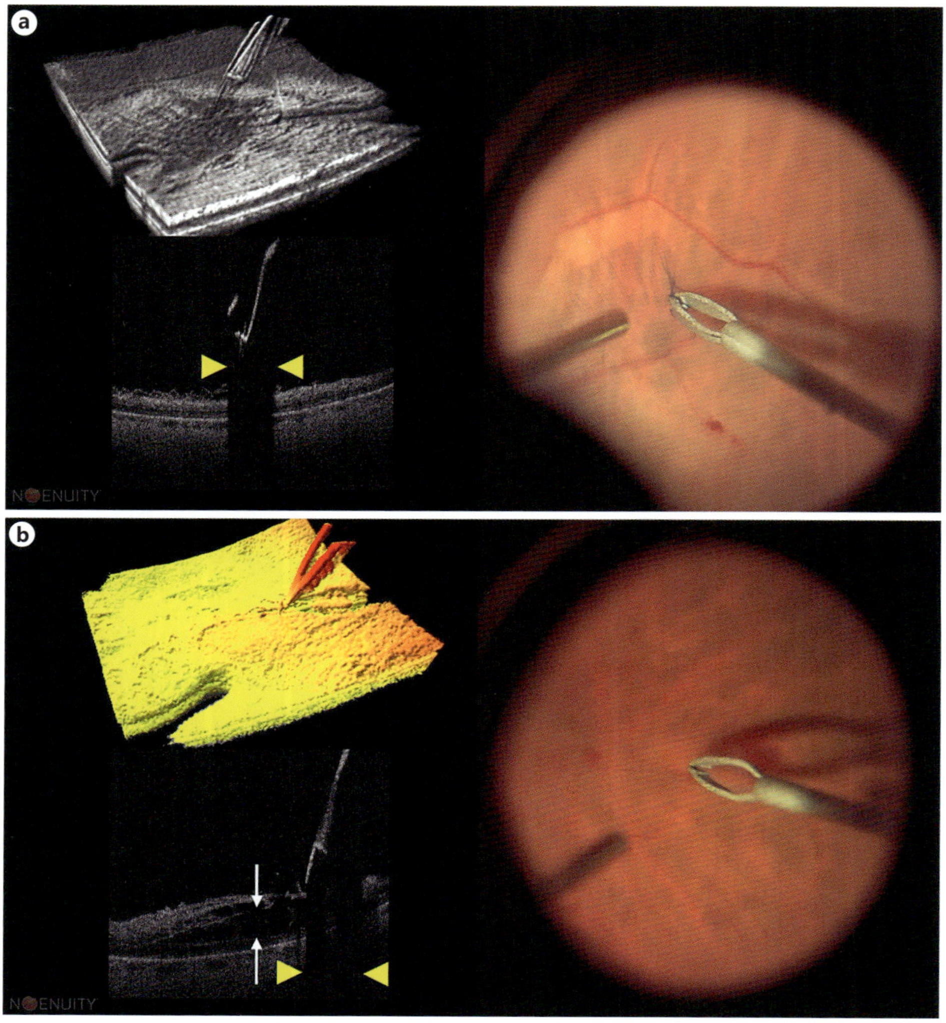

Fig. 3. Volumetric Investigational Intraoperative Microscope-Integrated OCT. Still frame intraoperative (**a**) grayscale and (**b**) colorized volumetric images from an investigational swept-source microscope-integrated optical coherence tomography (OCT) device developed at Duke University [14, 15] used during brilliant blue-assisted epiretinal membrane peels in two different cases. In each panel, the top left image is a 3D volumetric OCT scan of a region of interest determined by the surgeon, the bottom left image is a 2D OCT B-scan, and the right image shows the surgical field, captured using the Ngenuity 3D Visualization System. The yellow arrowheads highlight shadow artifacts on 2D OCT B-scans that appear posterior to metallic instruments such as internal limiting membrane forceps. Colorization is used to highlight more elevated areas (internal limiting membrane forceps in red) compared to less elevated areas (retina and epiretinal membrane in yellow). Note that the 2D OCT B-scan in (**b**) also demonstrates retinoschisis (white arrows) that is not as evident from the surgical field alone. The authors thank Jianwei D. Li and William Raynor for help with acquiring these images.

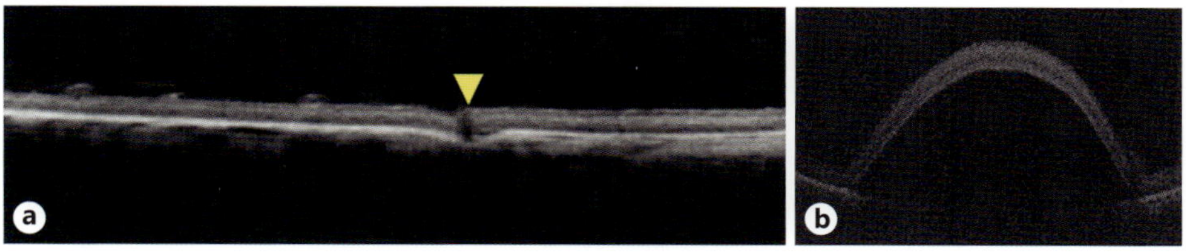

Fig. 4. Intraoperative OCT of subretinal bleb creation. Zeiss RESCAN 700 OCT 2D B-scans demonstrating retinal depression (arrowhead) (**a**) during retinotomy creation using a subretinal injection needle to facilitate subretinal bleb formation in a porcine eye (**b**).

retinal detachments, choroidal rupture with associated choroidal neovascularization, and subhyaloid or subretinal hemorrhage (Fig. 2b) [1]. In a case report of a 1-year-old infant with vitreous hemorrhage and fovea-involving sub-internal limiting membrane fibrotic consolidated hemorrhage in the setting of Terson syndrome, intraoperative OCT was used to guide careful dissection of the internal limiting membrane using a bent 30-G needle, as well as removal of the fibrotic material with internal limiting membrane forceps [54]. In patients with submacular hemorrhage, intraoperative OCT can be used to measure the thickness of the subretinal hemorrhage, identify associated underlying choroidal neovascularization, and guide subretinal injection of tissue plasminogen activator when surgical evacuation is preferred [55]. In cases associated with traumatic cataract requiring pars plana lensectomy, MIOCT can also be focused anteriorly to improve visualization of the anterior capsule and ensure its preservation during lensectomy [56].

Pediatric patients are an important target for intraoperative OCT-guided subretinal gene delivery for inherited retinal diseases. In Leber congenital amaurosis, it has been suggested that areas of preserved foveal or parafoveal microstructural anatomy as identified by OCT may be more likely to benefit from subretinal gene delivery [57]. Intraoperative OCT may thus be used to guide identification of the optimal delivery sites for gene therapy. Current protocols for subretinal gene delivery recommend pars plana vitrectomy followed by the induction of macular detachment via subretinal injection of balanced salt solution through a retinotomy, with subsequent subretinal delivery of a genetic vector [8]. MIOCT has been used in pediatric and adult patients to monitor the indentation and penetration of the neurosensory retina during subretinal bleb formation (Fig. 4a), visualize subretinal bleb formation (Fig. 4b) as well as the degree of reflux from the subretinal bleb back to the vitreous cavity, and identify the original subretinal bleb retinotomy site when proceeding with subretinal genetic vector injection [58, 59]. MIOCT has a particularly important role in assessing for potential complications such as inadvertent injection into the intraretinal or suprachoroidal space or iatrogenic creation of a macular hole [8]. In choroideremia, MIOCT has been reported to be useful in monitoring the direction of progression of subretinal injection to give the surgeon real-time feedback on how to avoid the overextension of areas of excessive retinal thinning or subretinal adhesions [60]. By offering high-resolution visualization of the extent of subretinal bleb formation, MIOCT can also enable the identification of adequate, albeit shallow, retinal detachment in the targeted delivery site, allowing precise targeting of subretinal gene therapy while minimizing excessive retinal stretching [60].

Future Considerations

To further expand the utility of MIOCT to pediatric vitreoretinal surgery, there has been interest in developing surgical instruments that are more compatible with MIOCT than traditional metallic instruments, which impair OCT visualization of underlying tissues due to shadowing and light scattering effects (Fig. 3) [61–64]. Surgical instruments made from silicone and plastic have been found to interfere less with OCT visualization of the underlying retina, but are not reusable and may have different mechanical properties from their metallic counterparts [61, 63, 64].

MIOCT offers the unique opportunity to incorporate intraoperative multimodal imaging into the diagnosis and management of pediatric vitreoretinal diseases. An investigational 100-kHz swept-source MIOCT angiography system has been shown to have potential in revealing subtle vascular changes in the posterior pole and midperiphery that may be difficult to distinguish on fluorescein angiography due to the small diameter of the involved vasculature and/or obscuration from adjacent fluorescein staining or leakage [4]. As OCT angiography technology improves, especially with respect to the ability to image the peripheral retina, rapid intraoperative OCT angiography imaging may offer unique insight into the etiology and optimal management of retinal vascular diseases requiring surgery for associated complications.

Research is actively ongoing into optimization of MIOCT technology to broaden its applications to pediatric and adult vitreoretinal surgery. The ideal MIOCT system should feature an imperceptible time lag between surgeon movement and OCT imaging, automated tracking [62] of moving surgical instruments, wide-field scanning of not only the area of interest but also more remote vitreous and retinal areas that may be impacted by surgical manipulations in the area of interest, and reproducible, high-resolution imaging through the level of the choroid. Investigational swept-source MIOCT prototypes with volumetric postprocessing technology developed at Duke [59, 65] and elsewhere [66] are enabling 4D-MIOCT imaging, or real-time volumetric and en face OCT superposition on the surgical field, which the surgeon can view either through the microscope oculars or on a separate magnified external display, such as Ngenuity (Alcon, Fort Worth, TX, USA). Topographic colorization of OCT structures and surgeon-controlled rotation of the viewing angle of OCT imaging using a joystick have been used to further enhance surgeon appreciation of the three-dimensional anatomy of the surgical field, increasing surgical safety and efficiency (Fig. 3b) [65, 67]. In addition, because OCT allows for the possibility of quantitative measurements, 4D-MIOCT systems coupled with quantitative postprocessing technology and robotic feedback systems may offer unprecedented surgical precision. As just one example of the potential power of quantification, researchers at Duke have developed methods of measuring subretinal bleb volume from real-time intraoperative OCT imaging, with the goal of enabling precise delivery of desired volumes of subretinal gene therapy [68, 69].

As with any novel technology, there is a learning curve to the incorporation of MIOCT into vitreoretinal surgery, and surgical case times may be increased, especially initially [7]. The ability to visualize retinal structural detail with MIOCT is also limited in the presence of significant cataract or other media opacity, as with any OCT system. Notwithstanding these limitations, it is our experience that MIOCT, and especially 4D-MIOCT, can significantly improve intraoperative visualization of vitreoretinal anatomy, and is an essential component of the pediatric vitreoretinal surgeon's toolkit. As MIOCT becomes more widely adopted in clinical practice, particularly in macular surgery and surgery requiring membrane peeling, we look forward to more publications on MIOCT-assisted surgical techniques and outcomes, as well as correlations between intraoperative anatomic findings and postoperative prognosis.

Conflict of Interest Statement

S.C.: None
A.T.: Heidelberg Engineering - research grant; Orbit Biomedical - research grant
L.V.: Alcon - consultant, research grant; Zeiss - research equipment; Heidelberg Engineering - research grant, research equipment.

Author Contributions

S.C., A.T., and L.V. fulfilled all of the following: (1) substantial contributions to the conception or design of the work; or the acquisition, analysis, or interpretation of data for the work; (2) drafting the work or revising it critically for important intellectual content; (3) final approval of the version to be published.

References

1 Scott AW, Farsiu S, Enyedi LB, Wallace DK, Toth CA: Imaging the infant retina with a hand-held spectral-domain optical coherence tomography device. Am J Ophthalmol 2009;147:364–373.e362.
2 Chong GT, Farsiu S, Freedman SF, et al: Abnormal foveal morphology in ocular albinism imaged with spectral-domain optical coherence tomography. Arch Ophthalmol 2009;127:37–44.
3 Dayani PN, Maldonado R, Farsiu S, Toth CA: Intraoperative use of handheld spectral domain optical coherence tomography imaging in macular surgery. Retina 2009;29:1457–1468.
4 Chen X, Viehland C, Carrasco-Zevallos OM, et al: Microscope-integrated optical coherence tomography angiography in the operating room in young children with retinal vascular disease. JAMA Ophthalmol 2017;135:483–486.
5 Carrasco-Zevallos OM, Keller B, Viehland C, et al: Live volumetric (4D) visualization and guidance of in vivo human ophthalmic surgery with intraoperative optical coherence tomography. Sci Rep 2016;6:31689.
6 Siebelmann S, Handel A, Matthaei M, Bachmann B, Cursiefen C: Microscope-integrated optical coherence tomography-guided drainage of acute corneal hydrops in keratoconus combined with suturing and gas-aided reattachment of Descemet membrane. Cornea 2019;38:1058–1061.
7 Runkle A, Srivastava SK, Ehlers JP: Microscope-integrated OCT feasibility and utility with the EnFocus System in the DISCOVER Study. Ophthalmic Surg Lasers Imaging Retina 2017;48:216–222.
8 Gregori NZ, Lam BL, Davis JL: Intraoperative use of microscope-integrated optical coherence tomography for subretinal gene therapy delivery. Retina 2019;39(Suppl 1):S9–S12.
9 Ehlers JP: Intraoperative optical coherence tomography: past, present, and future. Eye 2016;30:193–201.
10 Lu CD, Waheed NK, Witkin A, et al: Microscope-integrated intraoperative ultrahigh-speed swept-source optical coherence tomography for widefield retinal and anterior segment imaging. Ophthalmic Surg Lasers Imaging Retina 2018;49:94–102.
11 Viehland C, Keller B, Carrasco-Zevallos OM, et al: Enhanced volumetric visualization for real time 4D intraoperative ophthalmic swept-source OCT. Biomed Opt Express 2016;7:1815–1829.
12 Shen L, Carrasco-Zevallos O, Keller B, et al: Novel microscope-integrated stereoscopic heads-up display for intrasurgical optical coherence tomography. Biomed Opt Express 2016;7:1711–1726.
13 Figueiredo N, Talcott KE, Srivastava SK, et al: Conventional microscope-integrated intraoperative OCT versus digitally enabled intraoperative OCT in vitreoretinal surgery in the DISCOVER study. Ophthalmic Surg Lasers Imaging Retina 2020;51:S37–S43.
14 Viehland C, Dhalla AZ, Li JD, et al: Real time volumetric intrasurgical optical coherence tomography with 4D visualization of surgical maneuvers. Paper presented at SPIE BiOS 2020 Virtual Annual Meeting; March 9, 2020.
15 Vajzovic L, Viehland C, Li JD, et al: The next generation MIOCT system: real time volumetric intraoperative optical coherence tomography with 4D visualization of surgical maneuvers. Paper presented at American Society of Retinal Specialists 2020 Virtual Annual Meeting; July 24, 2020.
16 Grewal DS, Tran-Viet D, Vajzovic L, Mruthyunjaya P, Toth CA: Association of pediatric choroidal neovascular membranes at the temporal edge of optic nerve and retinochoroidal coloboma. Am J Ophthalmol 2017;174:104–112.
17 Ong SS, Hsu ST, Grewal D, et al: Appearance of pediatric choroidal neovascular membranes on optical coherence tomography angiography. Graefes Arch Clin Exp Ophthalmol 2020;258:89–98.
18 Chen X, Mangalesh S, Dandridge A, et al: Spectral-domain OCT findings of retinal vascular-avascular junction in infants with retinopathy of prematurity. Ophthalmol Retina 2018;2:963–971.
19 Mangalesh S, Bleicher ID, Chen X, et al: Three-dimensional pattern of extraretinal neovascular development in retinopathy of prematurity. Graefes Arch Clin Exp Ophthalmol 2019;257:677–688.
20 Zepeda EM, Shariff A, Gillette TB, et al: Vitreous bands identified by handheld spectral-domain optical coherence tomography among premature infants. JAMA Ophthalmol 2018;136:753–758.
21 Chavala SH, Farsiu S, Maldonado R, Wallace DK, Freedman SF, Toth CA: Insights into advanced retinopathy of prematurity using handheld spectral domain optical coherence tomography imaging. Ophthalmology 2009;116:2448–2456.
22 Lee AC, Maldonado RS, Sarin N, et al: Macular features from spectral-domain optical coherence tomography as an adjunct to indirect ophthalmoscopy in retinopathy of prematurity. Retina 2011;31:1470–1482.
23 Chen X, Prakalapakorn SG, Freedman SF, Vajzovic L, Toth CA: Differentiating retinal detachment and retinoschisis using handheld optical coherence tomography in stage 4 retinopathy of prematurity. JAMA Ophthalmol 2019;138:81–85.

24 Campbell JP, Nudleman E, Yang J, et al: Handheld optical coherence tomography angiography and ultra-wide-field optical coherence tomography in retinopathy of prematurity. JAMA Ophthalmol 2017;135:977–981.
25 Legocki AT, Zepeda EM, Gillette TB, et al: Vitreous findings by handheld spectral-domain oct correlate with retinopathy of prematurity severity. Ophthalmol Retina 2020;4:1008–1015.
26 Moshiri Y, Legocki AT, Zhou K, et al: Handheld swept-source optical coherence tomography with angiography in awake premature neonates. Quant Imaging Med Surg 2019;9:1495–1502.
27 Yonekawa Y, Thomas BJ, Drenser KA, Trese MT, Capone A Jr: Familial exudative vitreoretinopathy: spectral-domain optical coherence tomography of the vitreoretinal interface, retina, and choroid. Ophthalmology 2015;122:2270–2277.
28 Lee J, El-Dairi MA, Tran-Viet D, et al: Longitudinal changes in the optic nerve head and retina over time in very young children with familial exudative vitreoretinopathy. Retina 2019;39:98–110.
29 Lytvynchuk LM, Glittenberg CG, Ansari-Shahrezaei S, Binder S: Intraoperative optical coherence tomography assisted analysis of pars plana vitrectomy for retinal detachment in morning glory syndrome: a case report. BMC Ophthalmol 2017;17:134.
30 Makdoumi K, Crafoord S: A prospective long-term follow-up study of optic disc pit maculopathy treated with pars plana vitrectomy, drainage of subretinal fluid and peeling of internal limiting membrane. Acta Ophthalmol 2020;98:822–827.
31 Alsulaiman SM, Al-Abdullah AA, Alakeely A, et al: Macular hole-related retinal detachment in children with knobloch syndrome. Ophthalmol Retina 2020;4:498–503.
32 Shinoda H, Koto T, Fujiki K, Murakami A, Tsubota K, Ozawa Y: Clinical findings in a choroideremia patient who underwent vitrectomy for retinal detachment associated with macular hole. Jpn J Ophthalmol 2011;55:169–171.
33 Sinha MK, Chhablani J, Shah BS, Narayanan R, Jalali S: Surgical challenges and outcomes of rhegmatogenous retinal detachment in albinism. Eye 2016;30:422–425.
34 Abouammoh MA, Alsulaiman SM, Gupta VS, et al: Surgical outcomes and complications of rhegmatogenous retinal detachment in eyes with chorioretinal coloboma: the results of the KKESH International Collaborative Retina Study Group. Retina 2017;37:1942–1947.
35 Gopal L, Badrinath SS, Sharma T, et al: Surgical management of retinal detachments related to coloboma of the choroid. Ophthalmology 1998;105:804–809.
36 Hussain RM, Abbey AM, Shah AR, Drenser KA, Trese MT, Capone A Jr: Chorioretinal coloboma complications: retinal detachment and choroidal neovascular membrane. J Ophthalmic Vis Res 2017;12:3–10.
37 Yee P, Sevgi DD, Abraham J, et al: iOCT-assisted macular hole surgery: outcomes and utility from the DISCOVER study. Br J Ophthalmol 2020. doi: 10.1136/bjophthalmol-2020-316045.
38 Kumar JB, Ehlers JP, Sharma S, Srivastava SK: Intraoperative OCT for uveitis-related vitreoretinal surgery in the DISCOVER study. Ophthalmol Retina 2018;2:1041–1049.
39 Ehlers JP, Modi YS, Pecen PE, et al: The DISCOVER Study 3-year results: feasibility and usefulness of microscope-integrated intraoperative oct during ophthalmic surgery. Ophthalmology 2018;125:1014–1027.
40 Strampe MR, Kaehr MM, Carroll J, Kim JE: Intraoperative imaging of retained perfluorocarbon liquid using spectral domain optical coherence tomography. Retin Cases Brief Rep 2019;13:381–384.
41 Smith AG, Cost BM, Ehlers JP: Intraoperative OCT-assisted subretinal perfluorocarbon liquid removal in the DISCOVER Study. Ophthalmic Surg Lasers Imaging Retina 2015;46:964–966.
42 Agarwal A, Gupta V: Intraoperative optical coherence tomography and proportional reflux hydrodissection-guided pars plana vitrectomy for complex severe proliferative diabetic retinopathy. Indian J Ophthalmol 2020;68:177–181.
43 Gabr H, Chen X, Zevallos-Carrasco OM, et al: Visualization from intraoperative swept-source microscope-integrated optical coherence tomography in vitrectomy for complications of proliferative diabetic retinopathy. Retina 2018;38(Suppl 1):S110–S120.
44 Wykoff CC, Berrocal AM, Schefler AC, Uhlhorn SR, Ruggeri M, Hess D: Intraoperative OCT of a full-thickness macular hole before and after internal limiting membrane peeling. Ophthalmic Surg Lasers Imaging 2010;41:7–11.
45 Ehlers JP, Khan M, Petkovsek D, et al: Outcomes of intraoperative OCT-assisted epiretinal membrane surgery from the PIONEER Study. Ophthalmol Retina 2018;2:263–267.
46 Ferrone PJ, Chaudhary KM: Macular epiretinal membrane peeling treatment outcomes in young children. Retina 2012;32:530–536.
47 Bonnin S, Metge F, Guez A, Edelson C, Dureau P, Caputo G: Long-term outcome of epiretinal membrane surgery in young children. Retina 2016;36:558–564.
48 Cohn AD, Quiram PA, Drenser KA, Trese MT, Capone A Jr: Surgical outcomes of epiretinal membranes associated with combined hamartoma of the retina and retinal pigment epithelium. Retina 2009;29:825–830.
49 Benhamou N, Massin P, Spolaore R, Paques M, Gaudric A: Surgical management of epiretinal membrane in young patients. Am J Ophthalmol 2002;133:358–364.
50 Khaja HA, McCannel CA, Diehl NN, Mohney BG: Incidence and clinical characteristics of epiretinal membranes in children. Arch Ophthalmol 2008;126:632–636.
51 Banach MJ, Hassan TS, Cox MS, et al: Clinical course and surgical treatment of macular epiretinal membranes in young subjects. Ophthalmology 2001;108:23–26.
52 Wise GN: Clinical features of idiopathic preretinal macular fibrosis. Schoenberg Lecture. Am J Ophthalmol 1975;79:349–347.
53 Rothman AL, Folgar FA, Tong AY, Toth CA: Spectral domain optical coherence tomography characterization of pediatric epiretinal membranes. Retina 2014;34:1323–1334.
54 Hussain RM, Dubovy SR, Zhou XY, Schwartz SG, Villegas VM: Pars plana vitrectomy with intraoperative optical coherence tomography for sub-internal limiting membrane fibrosis excision in a child with Terson syndrome: surgical and pathological correlation. Am J Ophthalmol Case Rep 2019;15:100479.

55 Ehlers JP, Petkovsek DS, Yuan A, Singh RP, Srivastava SK: Intrasurgical assessment of subretinal tPA injection for submacular hemorrhage in the PIONEER study utilizing intraoperative OCT. Ophthalmic Surg Lasers Imaging Retina 2015;46:327–332.
56 Jayadev C, Dabir S, Vinekar A, Shah U, Vaid T, Yadav NK: Microscope-integrated optical coherence tomography: a new surgical tool in vitreoretinal surgery. Indian J Ophthalmol 2015;63:399–403.
57 Sumaroka A, Garafalo AV, Semenov EP, et al: Treatment potential for macular cone vision in leber congenital amaurosis due to CEP290 or NPHP5 mutations: predictions from artificial intelligence. Invest Ophthalmol Vis Sci 2019;60:2551–2562.
58 Vasconcelos HM Jr, Lujan BJ, Pennesi ME, Yang P, Lauer AK: Intraoperative optical coherence tomographic findings in patients undergoing subretinal gene therapy surgery. Int J Retina Vitreous 2020;6:13.
59 Vajzovic L, Sleiman K, Viehland C, et al: Four-dimensional microscope-integrated optical coherence tomography guidance in a model eye subretinal surgery. Retina 2019;39(Suppl 1):S194–S198.
60 Xue K, Groppe M, Salvetti AP, MacLaren RE: Technique of retinal gene therapy: delivery of viral vector into the subretinal space. Eye 2017;31:1308–1316.
61 Ehlers JP, Tao YK, Farsiu S, Maldonado R, Izatt JA, Toth CA: Integration of a spectral domain optical coherence tomography system into a surgical microscope for intraoperative imaging. Invest Ophthalmol Vis Sci 2011;52:3153–3159.
62 Hahn P, Carrasco-Zevallos O, Cunefare D, et al: Intrasurgical human retinal imaging with manual instrument tracking using a microscope-integrated spectral-domain optical coherence tomography device. Transl Vis Sci Technol 2015;4:1.
63 Ehlers JP, Srivastava SK, Feiler D, Noonan AI, Rollins AM, Tao YK: Integrative advances for OCT-guided ophthalmic surgery and intraoperative OCT: microscope integration, surgical instrumentation, and heads-up display surgeon feedback. PLoS One 2014;9:e105224.
64 Ehlers JP, Uchida A, Srivastava SK: Intraoperative optical coherence tomography-compatible surgical instruments for real-time image-guided ophthalmic surgery. Br J Ophthalmol 2017;101:1306–1308.
65 Seider MI, Carrasco-Zevallos OM, Gunther R, et al: Real-time volumetric imaging of vitreoretinal surgery with a prototype microscope-integrated swept-source OCT device. Ophthalmol Retina 2018;2:401–410.
66 Kolb JP, Draxinger W, Klee J, et al: Live video rate volumetric OCT imaging of the retina with multi-MHz A-scan rates. PLoS One 2019;14:e0213144.
67 Bleicher ID, Jackson-Atogi M, Viehland C, Gabr H, Izatt JA, Toth CA: Depth-based, motion-stabilized colorization of microscope-integrated optical coherence tomography volumes for microscope-independent microsurgery. Transl Vis Sci Technol 2018;7:1.
68 Hsu ST, Gabr H, Viehland C, et al: Volumetric measurement of subretinal blebs using microscope-integrated optical coherence tomography. Transl Vis Sci Technol 2018;7:19.
69 Sastry A, Li, D, Raynor W, et al: Microscope-integrated optical coherence tomography-guided volumetric measurements of subretinal blebs created by a novel suprachoroidal approach. Paper presented at the American Society of Retina Specialists 2020 Virtual Annual Meeting; July 26, 2020.

Lejla Vajzovic
Department of Ophthalmology, Duke University Eye Center
Duke University School of Medicine, 2351 Erwin Road
Durham, NC 27710 (USA)
lejla.vajzovic@duke.edu

Erratum

In the chapter by Cai et al. entitled "Pediatric Vitreoretinal Surgery and Integrated Intraoperative Optical Coherence Tomography" [Integrated Intraoperative Ocular Coherence Tomography for Pediatric Ocular Surgery. Dev Ophthalmol. Basel, Karger, 2021, vol 61, DOI 10.1159/000511818], the legend to Figure 1 was incomplete and should read as follows:

Fig. 1. Intraoperative OCT modalities. Representative spectral-domain OCT devices suitable for imaging pediatric patients in the operating room include: the commercially available portable handheld Bioptigen/Leica Envisu c2300 (**a**), investigational portable Heidelberg Spectralis Flex module (**b**), and commercially available MIOCT Zeiss RESCAN 700 system, coupled with the Zeiss OPMI LUMERA 700 surgical microscope (**c**). Written informed consent was obtained from participants prior to publication.

Integrated Intraoperative Ocular Coherence Tomography for Pediatric Ocular Surgery. Dev Ophthalmol. Basel, Karger, 2021, vol 61, pp 15–25
(DOI: 10.1159/000511818)

Published online: February 16, 2021

Integrated Intraoperative Ocular Coherence Tomography for Pediatric Ocular Surgery. Dev Ophthalmol. Basel, Karger, 2021, vol 61, pp 26–30 (DOI: 10.1159/000511819)

Integrated Intraoperative Optical Coherence Tomography in Strabismus Surgery

Parth R. Shah[a, b] Matthew S. Pihlblad[b]

[a]Sydney Children's and Prince of Wales Hospitals, Sydney, NSW, Australia; [b]UPMC Children's Hospital of Pittsburgh, Pittsburgh, PA, USA

Abstract

The advent of integrated intraoperative ocular coherence tomography (i^2OCT) has opened the door for safer more complex surgeries of the retina and cornea. However, to limit its use to just two subspecialties within ophthalmology is an opportunity lost for many other subspecialties. Here, we describe the use of i^2OCT in strabismus surgery. It can be used to identify extraocular muscles, especially in cases of strabismus reoperations, thereby augmenting the surgical technique. Its use to help train strabismus surgery is invaluable, allowing the trainee to understand the depth of the scleral pass during strabismus surgery. The authors describe these scenarios of training and augmenting the surgical technique.

Integrated intraoperative optical coherence tomography (i^2OCT) has a number of applications in strabismus surgery. The advantages of this technology include an improved safety profile, improved patient outcomes, and as a teaching tool. Many strabismus surgeons already use the operating microscope for the high magnification that it provides.

Scenarios

Scleral Pass Depth

The depth of scleral pass of the muscle sutures is of critical importance in strabismus surgery. A shallow pass can result in a slipped or "lost" muscle [1]. A full-thickness scleral pass resulting in globe perforation is associated with rare but serious complications, including retinal detachment and endophthalmitis [1–6].

Prior to the advent of i^2OCT, there was no technology to enable the strabismus surgeon to assess the depth of scleral suture passes. i^2OCT allows the surgeon to visualize the scleral pass in real time, as the suture is being guided through the sclera (Fig. 1). The depth can be monitored to ensure it is about 50% of the scleral thickness. The OCT is ori-

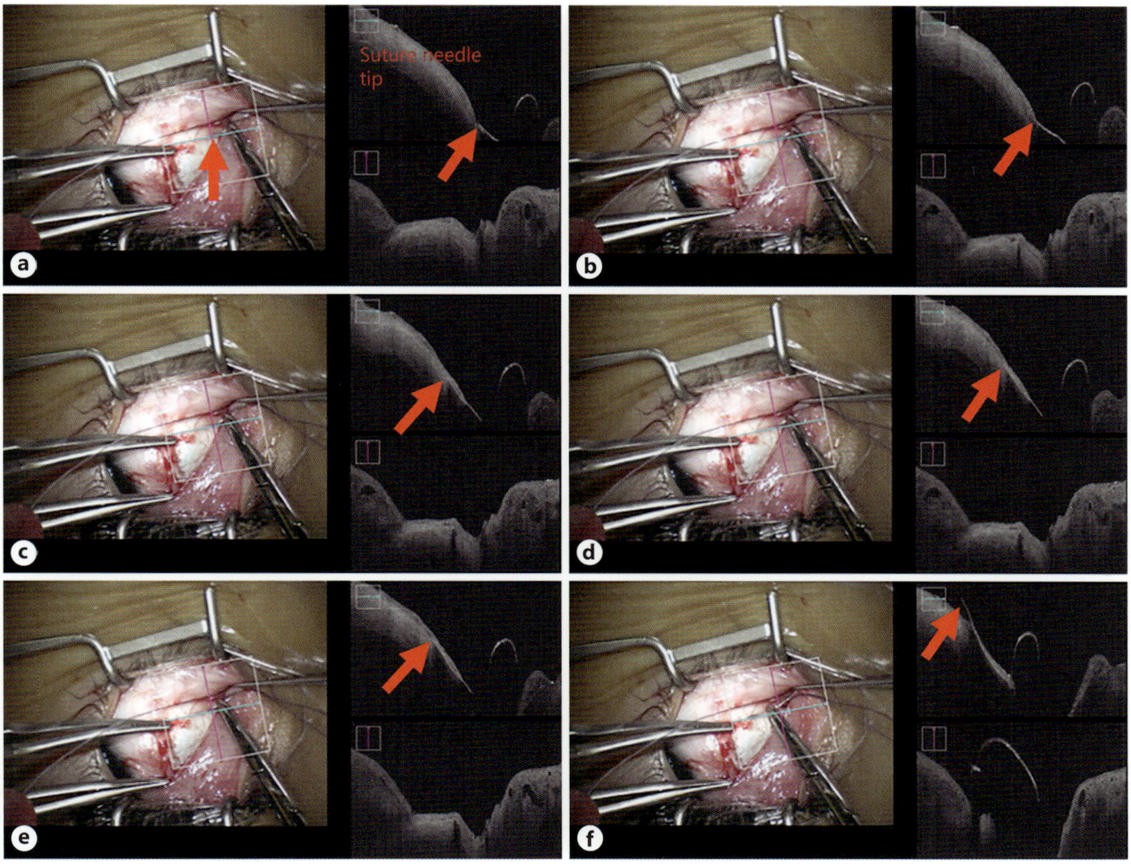

Fig. 1. a–f Assessing scleral suture pass in real time using i²OCT. Sequential snapshots of the surgical video are shown. The depth is relatively shallow, about 15% of scleral thickness.

ented so that one axis is perfectly parallel while the other is perpendicular to the suture needle.

Alternatively, i²OCT can be used after the suture has been passed through the sclera to confirm the depth is appropriate and safe. Watching the scleral pass in real time under the microscope oculars with OCT overlay can add an extra layer of complexity for a resident learning strabismus surgery. In these cases, the scleral pass depth in a training institution may be checked using i²OCT after the pass has already been made. Our team is incorporating i²OCT into the resident training program using animal eyes prior to surgery on real patients.

Knowing the true depth of scleral passes in relation to the clinical "feel" of the pass can help both novice and experienced surgeons appreciate the appropriate depth of the suture track. Figure 2 shows the scleral depth assessed using i²OCT after the suture has been passed. Both Figure 2a and b show an appropriate depth of about 50% scleral thickness. Note that in Figure 2a the cross-sectional scan (purple line) is not in the center of the scleral pass, therefore the depth appears less than 50%. Figure 2c shows a scleral pass which was very close to full thickness based on the i²OCT. This prompted the surgeon to perform a dilated fundus examination with scleral indenta-

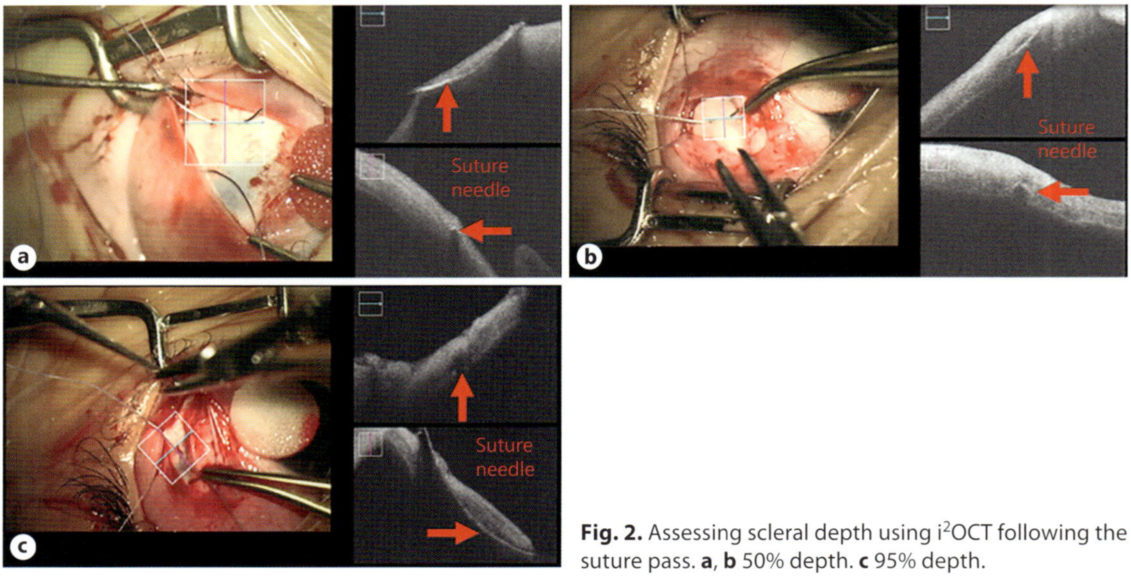

Fig. 2. Assessing scleral depth using i^{2}OCT following the suture pass. **a**, **b** 50% depth. **c** 95% depth.

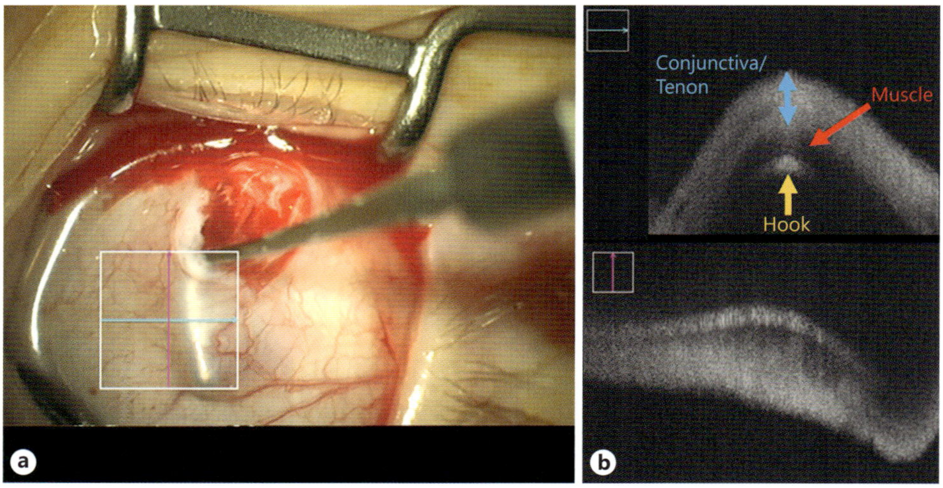

Fig. 3. Right eye, surgeon view sitting at the head. **a** The lateral rectus can be easily identified. **b** The lateral rectus muscle is hooked and can be clearly seen.

tion at the end of the case using indirect ophthalmoscopy. The suture was not seen, and there was no retinal hemorrhage or tear.

Identifying Extraocular Muscles

The utility of i^{2}OCT to identify insertions of extraocular muscles has been previously published [7–9]. This is particularly useful in cases where previous surgery has been performed and the muscle position is uncertain. It can guide appropriate conjunctival incisions and aid in surgical planning.

Figure 3a shows the anatomical landmarks and their appearance on i^{2}OCT. This can aid in appropriate conjunctival incision and muscle

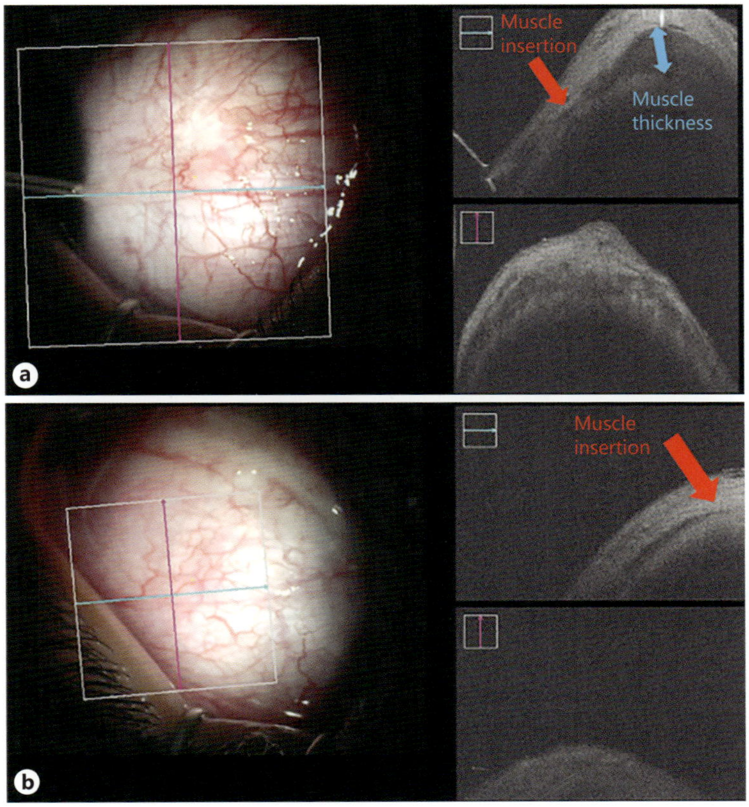

Fig. 4. Left eye, surgeon view sitting at the head. Red arrows show the rectus muscle insertions of the medial (**a**) and lateral (**b**) recti; the blue arrow shows the width of the rectus muscle previously resected. Conjunctival scarring is visible on the external view images, medial (**a**) more than lateral (**b**).

hooking (Fig. 3b), which has the benefit of reduced tissue trauma.

A previously operated strabismus patient is shown in Figure 4. The medial rectus is inserted a normal distance from the limbus with conjunctival scarring and thickening of the muscle which informed the surgeon that the muscle had a previous resection. The lateral rectus is noted to be far from the limbus (10.5 mm intraoperatively) with some mild conjunctival scarring, indicating to the surgeon that the lateral rectus had previously been recessed. The i^{2}OCT allows the surgeon to know the location of the muscles prior to any conjunctival incision and determine what surgery and what muscle(s) need to be operated on.

i^{2}OCT can be also used to reliably identify extraocular muscles and guide the injection of botulinum toxin (Fig. 5). This allows the surgeon to confidently deliver the drug directly into the muscle rather than injecting blindly, while also avoiding the need to open the conjunctiva. This has the theoretical benefit of reducing spread of the drug around the orbit to other extraocular muscles and the levator muscle.

Conclusion

i^{2}OCT is a useful tool for strabismus surgeons. The technology allows the surgeon to determine the location of the rectus muscle insertions prior to the start of surgery, helps with determining the placement of conjunctival incisions, gives feedback while hooking the muscle, can assess the depth and safety of the scleral pass, and determine the needle location during Botox injections. All of these benefits enhance the surgery, improve safety, and have important teaching implications for residents and fellows, along with strabismus surgeons.

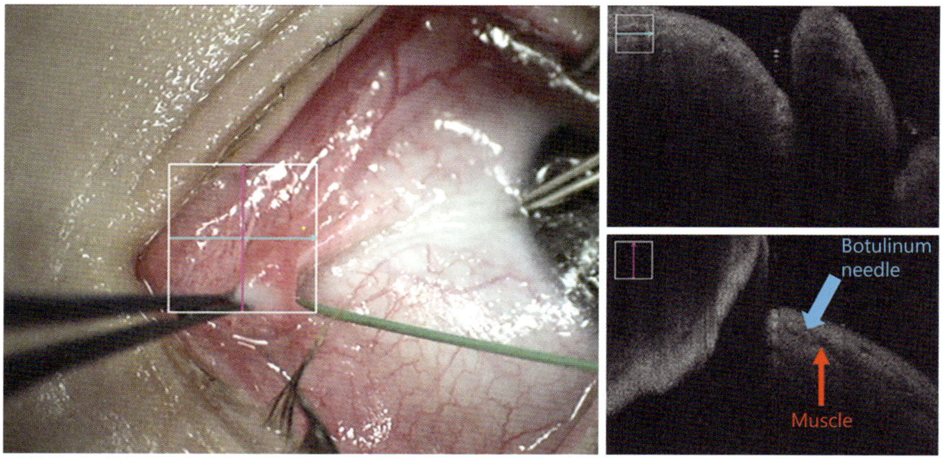

Fig. 5. i²OCT used to direct the injection of botulinum toxin into the right medial rectus muscle.

Conflict of Interest Statement

M.S.P. received grant support from the Knights Templar Eye Foundation and lecture honorariums from the World Society of Pediatric Ophthalmology and Strabismus.

Author Contributions

P.R.S. and M.S.P. fulfilled all of the following: (1) substantial contributions to the conception or design of the work; or the acquisition, analysis, or interpretation of data for the work; (2) drafting the work or revising it critically for important intellectual content; (3) final approval of the version to be published.

References

1 Bradbury JA, Taylor RH: Severe complications of strabismus surgery. J Aapos 2013;17:59–63.
2 Dang Y, Racu C, Isenberg SJ: Scleral penetrations and perforations in strabismus surgery and associated risk factors. J Aapos 2004;8:325–331.
3 Ing MR: Infection following strabismus surgery. Ophthalmic Surg 1991;22:41–43.
4 Morris RJ, Rosen PH, Fells P: Incidence of inadvertent globe perforation during strabismus surgery. Br J Ophthalmol 1990;74:490–493.
5 Noel LP, Bloom JN, Clarke WN, et al: Retinal perforation in strabismus surgery. J Pediatr Ophthalmol Strabismus 1997;34:115–117.
6 Simon JW, Lininger LL, Scheraga JL: Recognized scleral perforation during eye muscle surgery: incidence and sequelae. J Pediatr Ophthalmol Strabismus 1992;29:273–275.
7 Pihlblad MS, Troia A, Tibrewal S, et al: Pre-, intra-, and post-operative evaluation of extraocular muscle insertions using optical coherence tomography: a comparison of four devices. J Clin Med 2019;8:1732.
8 Pihlblad MS, Reynolds JD: Anterior segment optical coherence tomography of previously operated extraocular muscles. Am Orthopt J 2017;67:61–66.
9 Pihlblad MS, Erenler F, Sharma A, et al: Anterior segment optical coherence tomography of the horizontal and vertical extraocular muscles with measurement of the insertion to limbus distance. J Pediatr Ophthalmol Strabismus 2016;53:141–145.

Matthew S. Pihlblad
Children's Hospital of Pittsburgh, Children's Hospital Drive
45th & Penn Avenue, CHP Faculty Pavilion, Suite 5000
Pittsburgh, PA 15201 (USA)
matthew.pihlblad2@chp.edu

Published online: February 19, 2021

Integrated Intraoperative Ocular Coherence Tomography for Pediatric Ocular Surgery. Dev Ophthalmol. Basel, Karger, 2021, vol 61, pp 31–38 (DOI: 10.1159/000511820)

The Use of Optical Coherence Tomography as an Intraoperative Adjunct of Oculoplastic Surgery

Sabrina Mukhtar Jenny Yu

UPMC Children's Hospital of Pittsburgh, Pittsburgh, PA, USA

Abstract

The advent of integrated intraoperative optical coherence tomography (i[2]OCT) has opened the door for safer and more complex surgeries in the retina and cornea. However, to limit its use to just two subspecialties within ophthalmology is an opportunity lost for many other subspecialties. Here, we describe the use of i[2]OCT in oculoplastic surgery. It can be used in cases of severe symblepharon where the cornea is heavily involved, so that the surgeon is aware of the depth of the pannus when trying to remove it. It can also be used when the corneal planes are difficult to identify. In oculoplastic surgery the technology allows for identification of tissue planes when en face visualization is difficult due to developmental abnormalities and repeated surgeries. Our experience reflects some of the many uses of iOCT in ophthalmic surgery, highlighting its added value in surgical precision.

Like all fields in ophthalmology, oculoplastics is a visual field. Pathologies are either examined externally or by imaging when they are located deeper in the orbit. In the field of oculoplastics, the imaging modalities most commonly used for diagnostic purposes are undoubtedly computed tomography (CT) and magnetic resonance imaging [1]. These modalities are essential in making diagnoses and guiding treatment plans but are rarely used in real-time during surgical procedures as they pose a risk of excessive radiation exposure, especially in children.

The goal with any intraoperative imaging modality is to improve anatomical accuracy and the final procedural outcome without a significant increase in time or cost [2]. Two intraoperative modalities which are currently in use in the field of oculoplastics are stereotactic navigation (SNI) and ultrasound. The use of SNI during orbital surgeries has allowed the oculoplastic surgeon real-time feedback as to the location and efficacy of the procedures being performed by using bony landmarks, such as in orbital decompression for thyroid eye disease. However, because this procedure relies on preoperative imaging, it can be limited by changes in tissue positioning between the surgery and when the imaging was performed [3]. Similarly, ultrasound has many applications in ophthalmology, namely the B-scan and ultrasound biomicroscopy for assessing intraocular

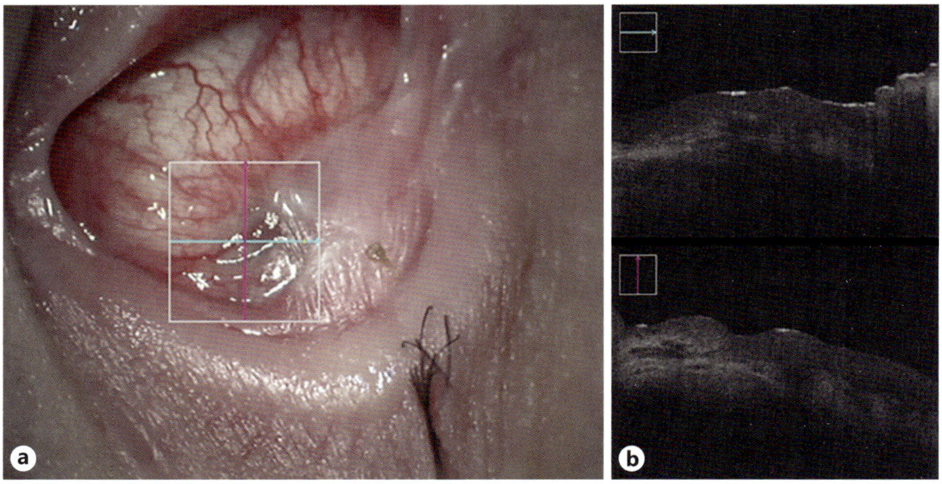

Fig. 1. Identification of tissue planes in obliterative conjunctival disease. **a** External photo of the right eye with obliteration of fornices and a difficult to identify tissue plane for surgical resection. **b** Intraoperative OCT with RESCAN 700 showing delineation between scar tissue and normal cornea and conjunctiva.

and orbital contents in a non-invasive, low cost way [4]. Unlike SNI and ultrasound, optical coherence tomography (OCT) has the potential to provide real-time feedback during eyelid procedures with significantly increased detail of soft tissue planes and pathology, thus potentially improving surgical outcomes.

OCT has been used in clinical applications since the mid-1990s with focus on preoperative planning and postoperative monitoring for ocular surgeries [5]. While initially mostly used for diagnostic purposes in the posterior segment, this imaging modality is now being used to image the ocular surface and anterior segment [6]. Interestingly, early studies of the use of intraoperative OCT (i^2OCT) have shown that i^2OCT provides superior resolution, is more cost effective, and can be easily incorporated into microscopes [7]. Many small retrospective cohorts have shown success with the use of i^2OCT in anterior and posterior segment surgeries. More recently, the DISCOVER and PIONEER studies have reported the success of i^2OCT in multi-surgeon prospective studies with various corneal and posterior segment surgeries [8, 9]. The real-time feedback influenced surgeon decision making to ensure better patient outcomes. While i^2OCT has been shown to be successful in intraocular surgeries, there are no reports investigating the use of this imaging modality in adnexal surgical interventions. While most oculoplastic procedures require only visualization using either surgical loupes or microscopes given the soft tissue depths, we aim to demonstrate the potential utility of i^2OCT in oculoplastics procedures, both eyelid and orbital, to improve surgical accuracy and clinical outcomes.

Scenarios

Case 1

A 2-year-old male with a complicated past ocular history including superficial keratitis of both eyes, right eye amblyopia, right eye corneal neovascularization, and a past medical history sig-

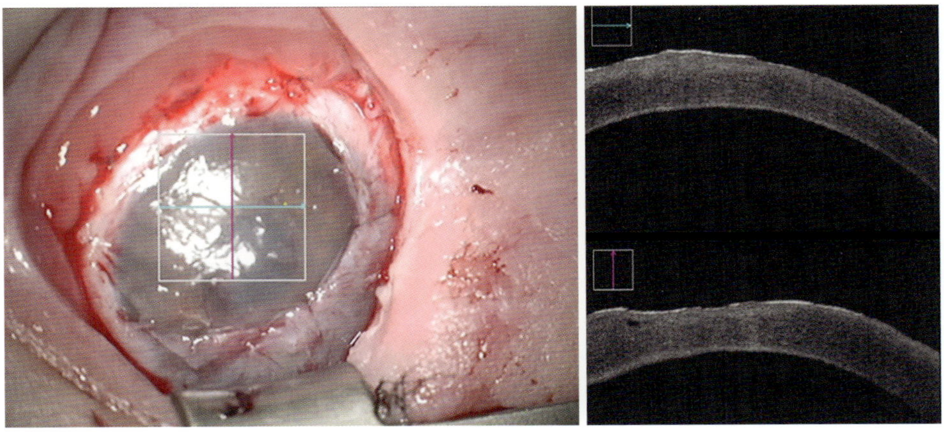

Fig. 2. Removal of pannus and scarring with an amniotic membrane placed.

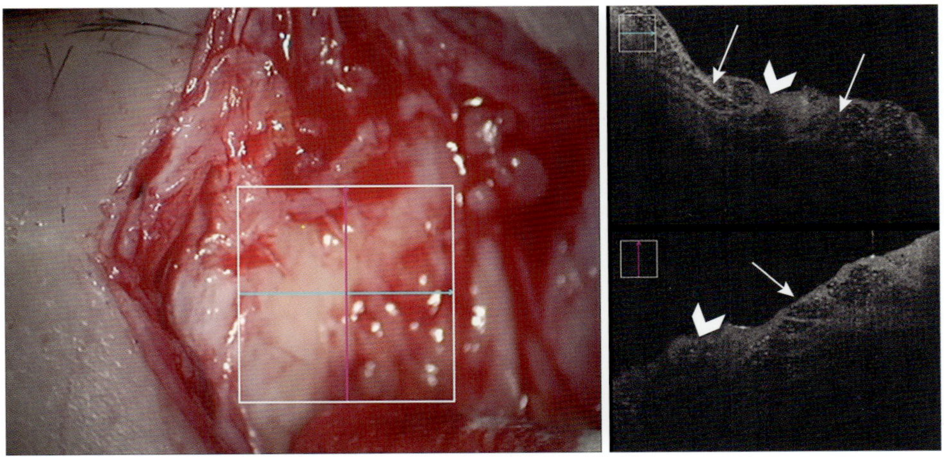

Fig. 3. Identification of scar tissue from the levator muscle using i^{2}OCT. The horizontal plane shows the area of scar tissue (white arrowhead) while the thin white arrows point to the levator muscle. The vertical plane similarly shows the levator muscle (thin white arrow) and also shows the scar tissue (white arrowhead).

nificant for toxic epidermal necrolysis syndrome presented to our institution for further evaluation of his obliterative conjunctival and corneal disease. His ocular surgical history was significant for several exams under anesthesia, multiple amniotic membrane transplants, and bevacizumab injections in both eyes. His medications included cyclosporine drops to both eyes twice a day and lubricating eye drops. Under our care he underwent several ophthalmologic procedures including right eye upper and lower fornices reconstruction, release of symblepharon, and dissection of overlying corneal pannus with the assistance of i^{2}OCT technology (Fig. 1). The i^{2}OCT allowed careful delineation of the pannus from the cornea and enabled a dissection of the pannus

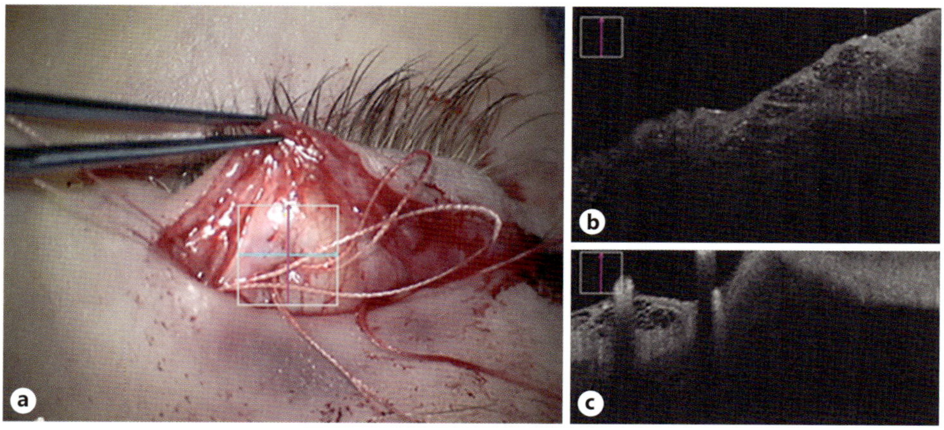

Fig. 4. Delineation of viable tissue from scar tissue with i^2OCT. **a** Intraoperative gross photo of the upper eyelid in a patient with congenital ptosis with residual scar tissue. The patient has a history of previous eyelid surgeries, and difficult to identify levator tissue. **b** Intraoperative OCT identifying the levator muscle. **c** Suture through the levator muscle.

off the cornea without disrupting the Bowman's membrane. An amniotic membrane was placed over the area freed of pannus (Fig. 2). In the immediate postoperative period, the patient had resolution of scar tissue and no surgical complications were noted. However, his inflammatory disease progressed, which led to right eye scleral thinning requiring a scleral tectonic patch graft. He is now 5 years old and his visual acuity is light perception in his right eye and hand motion in his left eye (the eye shown). His current medications include prednisolone 1% acetate every Monday, Wednesday, and Friday, erythromycin ointment to both eyes twice a day, and lubricating eye drops before bed. The appearance of both eyes was identical at presentation and, although he developed scarring, the vision in the eye that underwent removal of pannus is better than the eye that did not.

Case 2

A 15-year-old male with a past ocular history significant for a congenital left cranial nerve III palsy, strabismus, and diplopia was diagnosed with neurogenic ptosis with good levator muscle function at birth. His surgical history included a levator muscle resection in 2011, which was complicated by a chronic epithelial defect requiring reversal in 2012. He was followed for corneal surface disease, which was complicated by corneal scarring. Since his ptosis repair was reversed, his left visual axis continued to be obstructed. He was re-evaluated in 2018 for repair of complete ptosis. Due to the previous surgeries, he had residual scar tissue that was difficult to delineate with en face evaluation intraoperatively (Fig. 3). In order to better identify the levator muscle, i^2OCT was used to allow proper placement of a frontalis sling with silicone rods (Fig. 4). He did very well postoperatively and at his 7-month follow-up his ptosis was much improved, and the upper lid was approximated at the desired position. He did not suffer from any postoperative complications, including recurrence of corneal epithelial defects.

Case 3

A 6-year-old female with a past medical history significant for an 18p deletion and past ocular history of right congenital ptosis, limited leva-

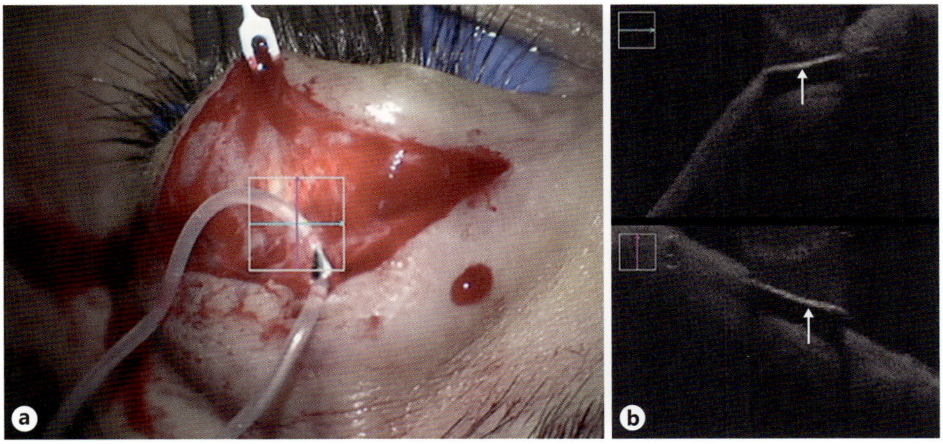

Fig. 5. Frontalis sling placement with i^2OCT. **a** External photograph of a patient with congenital ptosis requiring placement of a frontalis sling. **b** i^2OCT used to identify the correct tissue plane for frontalis sling placement which is in the levator muscle (white arrow).

tor muscle function, hypertropia, exotropia, and amblyopia presented to the oculoplastics service for surgical management. Her surgical history was significant for a right levator muscle resection just after birth. During her clinical course she continued to have bilateral ptosis, right greater than left. The right lid resided right over the visual axis with an MRD1 of 0.5 mm and left MRD1 of 1 mm at her preoperative evaluation. She underwent frontalis sling placement in the right eye at the age of 5 years with the assistance of i^2OCT (Fig. 5). It is very important to ensure that the slings are placed in the correct tissue plane. In Figure 5 the silicone slings are in the levator muscle (white arrow) as they should be. At her postoperative visits both surgeon and parents were happy with the lid positioning of her right eye and no complications were noted.

Case 4

A 15-year-old male with a past ocular history significant for cranial nerve III palsy, ptosis, and exposure keratopathy of the left eye was evaluated for a corneal neurotization for his neurotrophic cornea. His exam on presentation was significant for absent sensation of the lower two-thirds and reduced sensation of the upper third of the left cornea and scarring from previous exposure keratopathy. With a multi-disciplinary effort, the patient underwent a corneal neurotization procedure. His sural nerve was harvested and coapted to the right supratrochlear nerve; the graft was then passed through to the left upper eyelid crease via a subcutaneous tunnel through the glabellar region (Fig. 6). The sural nerve graft was passed into the subconjunctival space where it was divided into 5 fascicles, which were then sutured around the limbus of the left eye. The use of i^2OCT was integral in graft identification and securing of the sural nerve around the limbus (Fig. 7). At follow-up visits the patient complained of pain and numbness in his forehead and leg which were from the nerve harvest and implantation. At his 6-month follow-up his vision had improved significantly and he did have sensation in the superior temporal quadrant of the left cornea. No complications were noted from i^2OCT use.

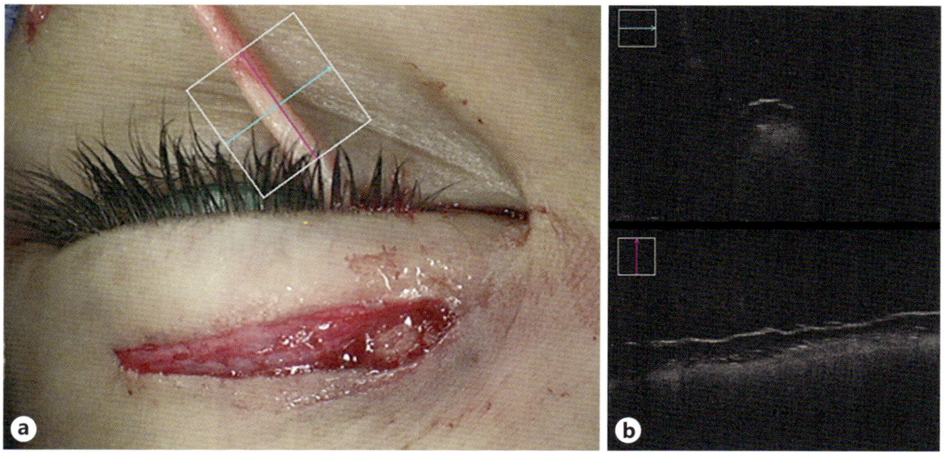

Fig. 6. Sural nerve identification for transposition through a left eyelid crease. **a** External photograph of the sural nerve after being passed through the left eyelid crease, ready for division of fascicles. **b** i^{2}OCT with horizontal and vertical cross-sections to help better identify fascicles for nerve transplantation.

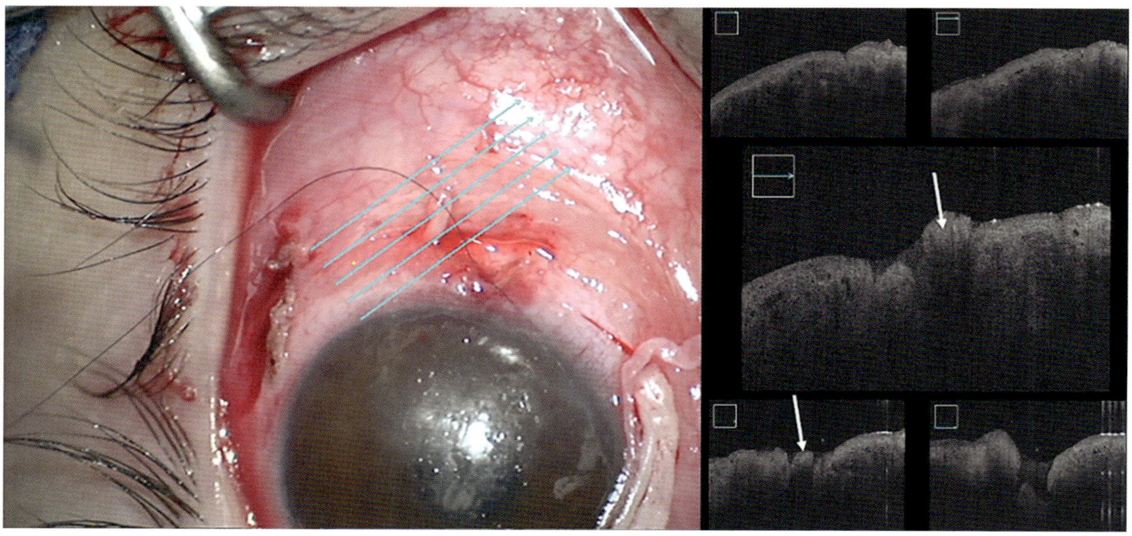

Fig. 7. Placement of sural nerve fascicles around the limbus. The fascicle can be seen in the cross-section (white arrows).

Discussion

The use of i^2OCT is a nascent and emerging field that is causing paradigm shifts in ophthalmic surgical interventions. A limitation of en face imaging of the surgical field through a microscope is the limited depth perception and visualization of subsurface anatomy; however, i^2OCT helps overcome this. The key technological developments that facilitated the use of OCT in the operating rooms include the use of handheld OCT probes and microscope-integrated OCT [10]. Given that the use of i^2OCT is a fairly innovative practice, only two prospective studies have been published thus far. The DISCOVER study, a multi-surgeon investigational study, aimed to better understand the feasibility and utility of a microscope-integrated i^2OCT (RESCAN700). During this study, there were no reports of the i^2OCT interfering with surgery, 69% of the surgeons preferred the real-time feedback, and in 36% of posterior segment surgeries real-time feedback changed surgeon decision making [8]. Similarly, in the PIONEER study a prospective, consecutive case series investigated a microscope mounted system. In 29% of lamellar keratoplasty procedures, for example, the surgeon believed a graft was entirely apposed, but i^2OCT showed persistent fluid resulting in additional manipulations, and in 48% of cases where surgeons were unsure regarding apposition, i^2OCT showed persistent fluid, again affecting surgical management intraoperatively [9]. The advantages for i^2OCT include the ability to better visualize tissue planes ultimately resulting in increased surgical success.

Our case series described above appears to be the first to use i^2OCT technology in oculoplastics procedures. As evidenced in the cases above, this imaging modality is especially useful in instances where normal anatomy cannot be identified by simple inspection of tissues due to either a disease process, abnormal development, or previous surgeries. While more experienced surgeons can rely on other queues for identifying and dissecting through challenging tissue planes, the availability of the i^2OCT technology can help trainees and newer surgeons to gain confidence as they develop surgical memory for these dissections. The use of i^2OCT in guiding and improving surgeon decision making would improve patient outcomes overall.

The limitations of i^2OCT include increased operating room time which can translate into higher costs for patients. The median time of surgery can increase from 0.4 to 26.7 min, depending on surgeon and operating room staff training [9]. Neither the DISCOVER nor PIONEER trials showed adverse effects specifically relating to i^2OCT use; however, it would be prudent to address the potential infection risk as one is placing a non-sterile device proximal to the surgical field. Furthermore, the handheld device does not provide true real-time feedback as the OCT must be moved into position to obtain scans. In our study specifically there was a small sample size, so we are unable to extrapolate the success to all oculoplastic surgeries. Additionally, the current focal length is ideal for intraocular surgical interventions and not the more anteriorly focused soft tissue of eyelid procedures, nor the depth of focus useful in orbital surgeries at this time. Even so, with the current modules not intended for oculoplastics use, the real-time feedback with its current en face resolution has proven utility in our surgical cases. There exists potential for the i^2OCT software modules to be paired/integrated with other microscopes of varying depth of focus that could allow it to operate similarly to the intraoperative CT guidance currently used in deeper orbital planes. While CT has better resolution, the tradeoff with i^2OCT is the lack of radiation exposure, which is of clinical importance in the pediatric population.

The i^2OCT has potential for image guidance in oculoplastics surgeries. Improved resolution and increased depth of focus can help delineate surgical planes in the various compartments of the orbit. The technology does have a learning curve, but its availability can add value to more challenging cases, as stated above. It also adds real-time feedback in the training of residents and fellows intraoperatively to improve their surgical memory. The use of the technology in the various oculoplastic procedures will help to further elucidate its potential over time.

Author Contributions

S.M. and J.Y. fulfilled all of the following: (1) substantial contributions to the conception or design of the work; or the acquisition, analysis, or interpretation of data for the work; (2) drafting the work or revising it critically for important intellectual content; (3) final approval of the version to be published.

Conflict of Interest Statement

The authors have nothing to disclose.

References

1 Cetinkaya A: Update on imaging techniques in oculoplastics. Saudi J Ophthalmol 2012;26:357–364.
2 Collyer J: Stereotactic navigation in oral and maxillofacial surgery. Br J Oral Maxillofac Surg 2010;48:79–83.
3 Millar MJ, Maloof AJ: The application of stereotactic navigation surgery to orbital decompression for thyroid-associated orbitopathy. Eye 2009;23:1565–1571.
4 Abhidnya S, Meel R, Pushker N, Bajaj MS: Ultrasound biomicroscopy image patterns in normal upper eyelid and congenital ptosis in the Indian population. Indian J Ophthalmol 2018;66:383–388.
5 Wilkins JR, Puliafito CA, Hee MR, Duker JS, Reichel E, Coker JG, Schuman JS, Swanson EA, Fujimoto JG: Characterization of epiretinal membranes using optical coherence tomography. Ophthalmology 1996;103:2142–2150.
6 Venkateswaran N, Galor A, Wang J, Karp CL: Optical coherence tomography for ocular surface and corneal diseases: a review. Eye Vis 2018;5:13.
7 Brezinski ME, Tearney GJ, Boppart SA, Swanson EA, Southern JF, Fujimoto JG: Optical biopsy with optical coherence tomography: feasibility for surgical diagnostics. J Surg Res 1997;71:32–40.
8 Ehlers JP, Goshe J, Dupps WJ, Kaiser PK, SIng RP, Gans R, et al: Determination of feasibility and utility of microscope integrated optical coherence tomography during ophthalmic surgery: the DISCOVER study and RESCAN results. JAMA Ophthalmol 2015;133:1124–1132.
9 Ehlers JP, Dupps WJ, Kaiser PK, Goshe J, SIngh RP, Petkovsek D, et al: The prospective intraoperative and perioperative ophthalmic imaging with optical coherence tomography (PIONEER) study: 2 year result. Am J Ophthalmol 2014;158:999–1007.
10 Carrasco-Zevallos OM, Viehland C, Keller B, Draelos M, Kuo AN, Toth CA, Izatt JA: Review of intraoperative optical coherence tomography: technology and applications. Biomed Opt Express 2017;8:1607–1637.

Jenny Yu
Children's Hospital of Pittsburgh, Children's Hospital Drive
45th & Penn Avenue, CHP Faculty Pavilion, Suite 5000
Pittsburgh, PA 15201 (USA)
yuj3@upmc.edu

Published online: February 16, 2021

Integrated Intraoperative Ocular Coherence Tomography for Pediatric Ocular Surgery. Dev Ophthalmol. Basel, Karger, 2021, vol 61, pp 39–44 (DOI: 10.1159/000511816)

Integrated Intraoperative Optical Coherence Tomography in Pediatric Glaucoma Surgery

Amgad Eldib Sarah Janczewski Ken K. Nischal

UPMC Children's Hospital of Pittsburgh, Pittsburgh, PA, USA

Abstract

The advent of integrated intraoperative optical coherence tomography (i^{2}OCT) has opened the door for safer and more complex surgeries in the retina and cornea. However, to limit its use to just two subspecialties within ophthalmology is an opportunity lost for many other subspecialties. Here, we describe the use of i^{2}OCT in pediatric glaucoma surgery. It can be used to identify Schlemm's canal, Barkan's membrane, demonstrate the corneal pathology in Haab's striae, and iris hypoplasia in cases of Axenfeld-Rieger anomaly. It can help identify drainage blebs that are filtering and those that are not, and identify successful drainage tube flushing. It has also been used to identify a ligating suture effect on a drainage tube. We describe these scenarios in relation to training and augmenting surgical techniques.

Pediatric glaucoma surgery can be fraught with complications such as hypotony, hemorrhage, and endophthalmitis often due to tissue elasticity, causing wounds to gape, causing overdrainage, bleeding, and ingress of possible infective agents. Integrated intraoperative optical coherence tomography (i^{2}OCT) helps flatten the learning curve, giving surgeons the ability to assess barely visible or transparent structures in the anterior segment of the eye [1]. i^{2}OCT provides high-resolution images of these structures with the added advantage of its non-contact technique [2].

So far in the literature i^{2}OCT has been used in glaucoma for diagnostic purposes where it has allowed the visualization of anterior segment abnormalities and morphological changes during examinations under anesthesia [2]. Its use has also been described in glaucoma surgeries. Some of these included the monitoring of the morphological changes of Schlemm's canal during canaloplasty, lysis of peripheral anterior synechiae, trabeculectomy, Ahmed valve implantation, needling of drainage blebs, and monitoring of microcystoid conjunctival spaces [2].

i^{2}OCT could mitigate the difficulties and risks with some glaucoma procedures. It allows the accurate assessment of the scleral thickness in trab-

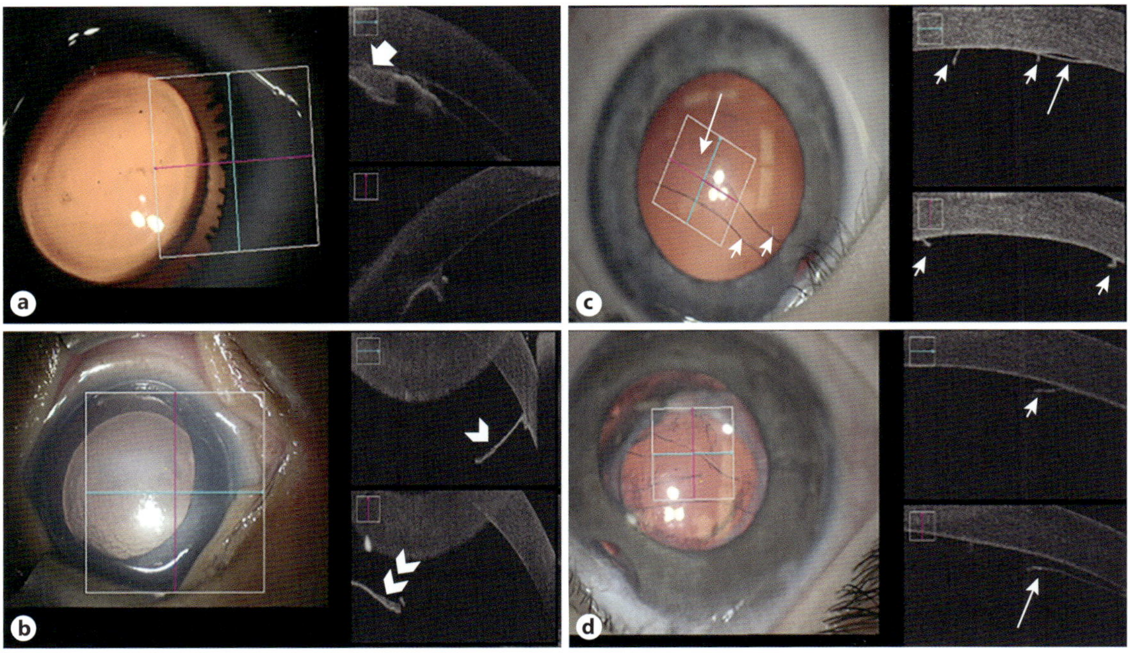

Fig. 1. a The remnants of the iris in a case of iris hypoplasia and illustrating the extent of iridocorneal adhesion (thick white arrow). **b** Scan in a patient with a known Axenfeld-Rieger anomaly and glaucoma demonstrating iris hypoplasia; complete absence of iris stroma (single white chevron) and partial absence of iris stroma (double white chevron). **c** A patient with glaucoma and a scan through Haab's striae demonstrating the breaks in Descemet's membrane (edges of breaks: short thin white arrows) and adjacent detachments (long thin white arrows). **d** Another scan in a different patient with glaucoma showing the Descemet's membrane breaks (short thin white arrow) in glaucoma with Descemet's membrane detachment (long thin white arrow).

eculectomy procedures in patients with thin sclera and more precise scleral flap lifting [1]. This would potentially reduce the chances of perforation with choroidal prolapse [1].

i²OCT has allowed direct monitoring and precise placement of surgical instruments in glaucoma procedures which might have been performed blindly in the past. This was more evident in cases that had trabeculectomy and developed an encapsulated bleb requiring needling of the bleb. It has also allowed improvement of the quality of glaucoma procedures and contributed greatly to the training of surgeons in the operative room [1, 3].

Here, we add our experience with diagnosis, teaching, and therapeutic surgical delivery of i²OCT in pediatric glaucoma. We will describe our experience using the surgical microscope (Zeiss, Jena, Germany) combined with an SD-OCT (RESCAN 700, Zeiss) which has a wavelength of 840 nm and a scanning speed of 27,000 A-scans per second.

Teaching

i²OCT not only allows real-time visualization of intraocular structures that are barely visible, but also an appreciation of their relations to surrounding tissues. Important examples are demonstrating that Haab's striae are not only breaks in the Descemet membrane but can be accompanied by detachments in the Descemet membrane, which are likely more common than reported [4] (Fig. 1c, d).

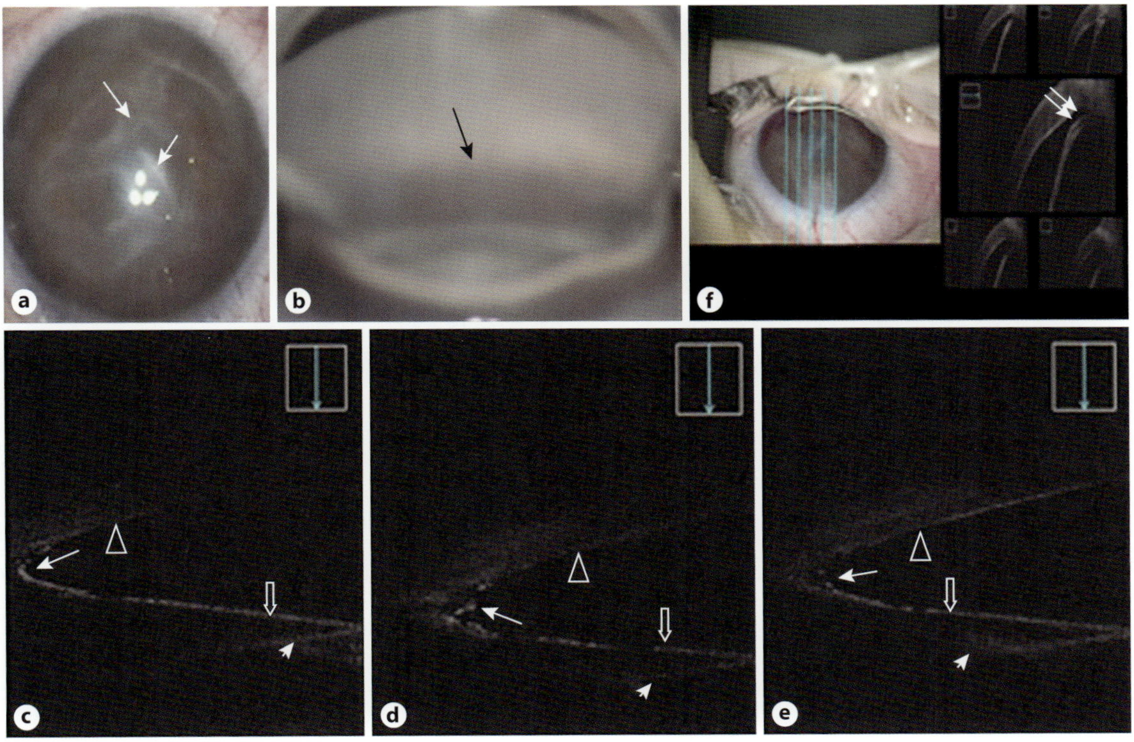

Fig. 2. This child with congenital glaucoma shows Haab's striae (**a**, white arrows) and shows anomalous tissue in the angle on gonioscopy (**b**, black arrow). **c–e** The integrated intraoperative OCT shows tissue in the angle visible (thin white arrow). Descemet membrane is seen and is indicated by the white triangle. The hypoplastic iris is shown by the long thick white arrow. The lens is indicated by the white arrowhead. **f** The picture following goniotomy with the tissue seen in **c–e** no longer present (double thin white arrow). Traditionally, this tissue seen in the angle is referred to as Barkan's membrane.

Demonstrating iris hypoplasia with i^2OCT allows an understating that the iris stroma can be partially or completely absent (Fig. 1a, b). This is not always appreciated in a child at the slit lamp, but during anesthesia the clinical suspicion can be confirmed. Confirmation of iridocorneal adhesion is also easily demonstrated (Fig. 1a). Keratolenticular adhesions can also of course be demonstrated very easily. Angle surgery is one of the surgeries used to treat congenital glaucoma. There is a membrane in the angle that hooks up the iris root and obscures the drainage angle. Incising this tissue allows better drainage of aqueous humor and control of glaucoma. This tissue was first described by Barkan [5] in 1955 and confirmed by Worst [6] in 1968 when it was then termed as Barkan's membrane. Whatever the nature of this tissue, we have used i^2OCT in conjunction with a direct gonioscope to image this prior to goniotomy. Again, this ability is invaluable when teaching fellows and residents (Fig. 2).

Diagnosis

In our practice, i^2OCT has become a fundamental diagnostic tool in patients with glaucoma. One important example is when a decision has

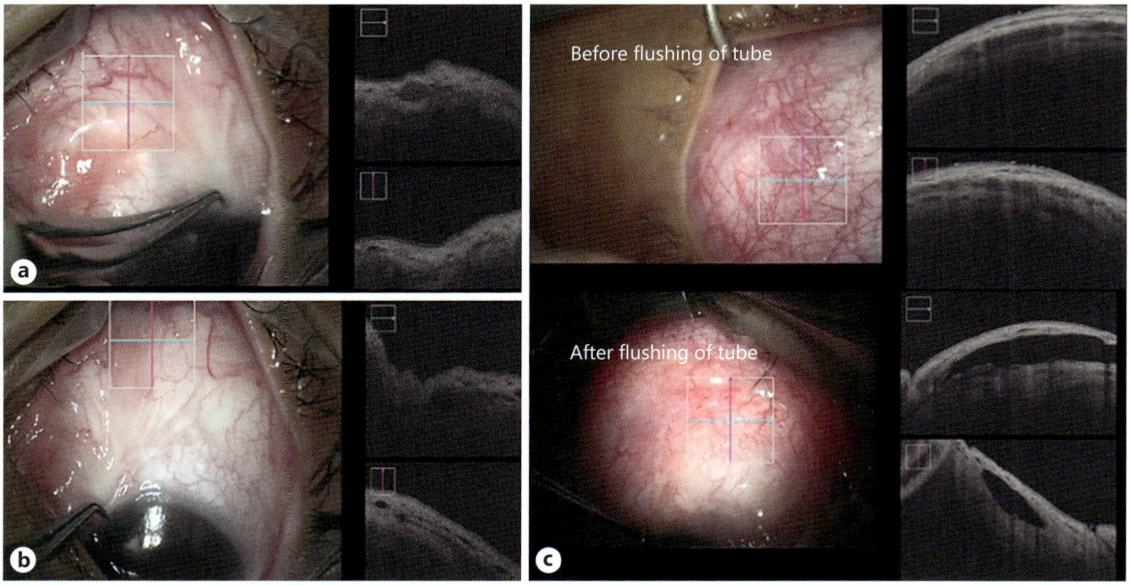

Fig. 3. a Scan through a trabeculectomy bleb demonstrating inadequate drainage evident by the low number and small size of subconjunctival microcystic spaces. **b** The same patient after successful ocular digital massage evident through the increased number and size of subconjunctival microcystic aqueous spaces. **c** A different patient with an Ahmed tube but inadequate drainage proven by OCT as illustrated by the very few microcystic spaces which, after flushing of the tube, show an increase in size, with successful re-establishment of aqueous drainage through the Ahmed tube into the subconjunctival space.

to be made as to whether a drainage bleb, either after trabeculectomy or following Ahmed tube implant, is still draining or has the potential to drain. In these circumstances using the detection of the number and size of conjunctival microcystic spaces allows surgeons to monitor and then, if necessary, modulate the drainage bleb. In a successful and patent drainage passage, multiple subconjunctival microcystic spaces could be easily seen. However, in cases where aqueous drainage into the subconjunctival space is reduced or absent, the number and size of the microcystic spaces is also absent or barely seen. During exam under anesthesia the blebs can be imaged, and if drainage is deemed inadequate ocular massage is performed to see the effect on the drainage bleb. If there is insufficient drainage seen despite ocular massage, then either bleb needling or tube flush can be performed. The presence of a Tenon's cyst can be detected too, which would necessitate a bleb fenestration or needling (Fig. 3).

Therapy

i^{2}OCT has helped flatten the learning curve of glaucoma surgery. It has allowed real-time visualization of the different ocular structures and accurate instrument placement during surgical procedures. Here, we will add some examples from our experience in which i^{2}OCT was very valuable in glaucoma surgical procedures.

i^{2}OCT has been described as very useful in trabeculectomy procedures. It allows the more precise fashioning and lifting of the scleral flap, espe-

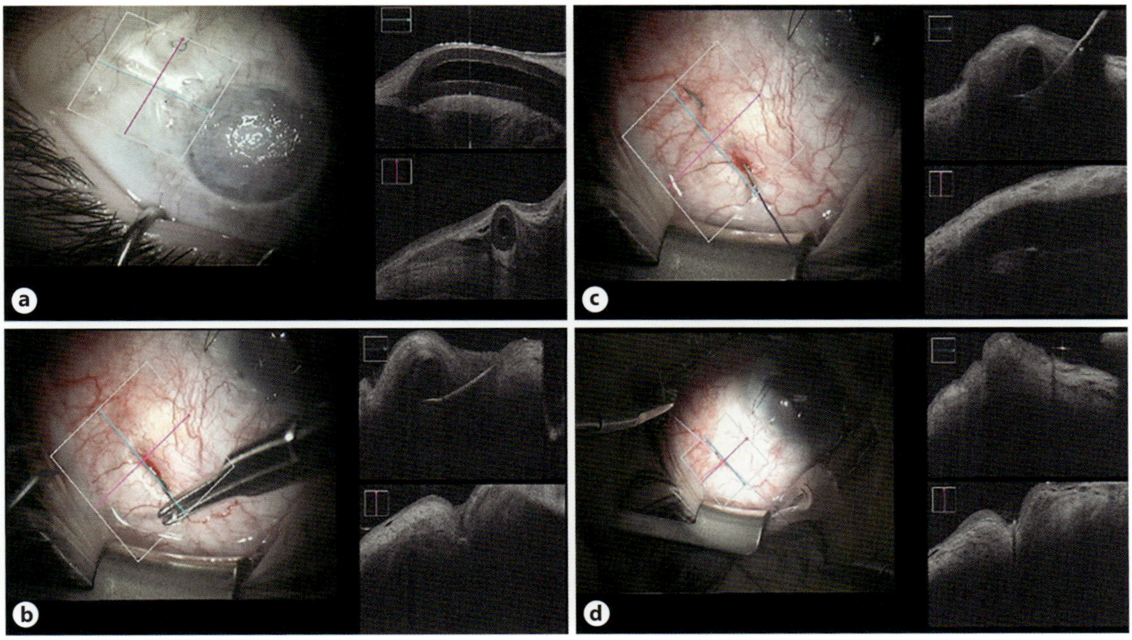

Fig. 4. a A patient with an Ahmed tube for glaucoma and scans showing the patency of the tube and its safe entry into the eye in a case with opaque cornea. **b** A different patient undergoing tying of an Ahmed tube. Scans showing the position of the needle in relation to the tube during initiation of the pass. **c** The same patient with scans showing the relation between the needle and the tube after the completion of pass of the needle. **d** A different scan in the same patient after tying down of the tube showing the occlusion of the lumen of the tube.

cially in cases that would otherwise be more difficult, such as those with thin sclera.

We would also like to add our experience with its use during the implantation of glaucoma drainage devices, such as the Ahmed drainage device. Placing the tube can be difficult in situations where the cornea is opaque or cloudy, often due to glaucoma, and especially in cases of pediatric corneal transplant. i^{2}OCT allows some visualization of the length of the intraocular portion of the tube and its relation to the surrounding structures. Assuring the tube was not in contact with the crystalline lens or the corneal endothelium is possible immediately after shunt placement. Any necessary adjustment of the tube length and position can be made if necessary (Fig. 4a).

On the other hand, excessive drainage in cases with tube implants is another situation where i^{2}OCT proved to be very valuable. Tying the tube was possible without dissecting the conjunctiva overlying it, which was previously necessary to visualize the tube. Tracking of the needle during the procedure made it less challenging. i^{2}OCT allowed the surgeon to ensure passage of the suturing needle deep into the tube without inadvertently entering the tube or penetrating the sclera. The change in configuration of the tube after tying compared to before allows the surgeon to assess the definite reduction in tube diameter (Fig. 4b–d). This can also be used when placing a tube to ensure either complete occlusion or partial occlusion depending on the case being treated.

Conflict of Interest Statement

K.K.N. has received honoraria from Carl Zeiss Meditech Inc. and is on the advisory board for Nevakar Inc.

Author Contributions

A.E., S.J., and K.K.N. fulfilled all of the following: (1) substantial contributions to the conception or design of the work; or the acquisition, analysis, or interpretation of data for the work; (2) drafting the work or revising it critically for important intellectual content; (3) final approval of the version to be published.

References

1 Stanzel BV, Gagalick A, Brinkmann CK, et al: Intraoperative OCT in der ophthalmologischen Mikrochirurgie. Ophthalmologe 2016;113:435–442.

2 Siebelmann S, Bachmann B, Lappas A, et al: Intraoperative optische Kohärenztomographie bei hornhaut- und glaukomchirurgischen Eingriffen. Ophthalmologe 2016;113:646–650.

3 Dada T, Angmo D, Midha N, et al: Intraoperative optical coherence tomography guided bleb needling. J Ophthalmic Vis Res 2016;11:452–454.

4 Mandal AK, Gothwal VK: Pre-Descemet's hematoma in a patient of congenital glaucoma with Descemet's detachment: a unique form of hemorrhage. Ophthalmic Surg Lasers 2000;31:427–428.

5 Barkan O: Pathogenesis of congenital glaucoma. Gonioscopic and anatomic observation of the angle of the anterior chamber in the normal eye and in congenital glaucoma. Am J Ophthailnol 1955;40:1–11.

6 Worst JGF: Congenital glaucoma. Remarks on the aspect of chamber angle: ontogenic and pathogenic background and mode of action of goniotomy. Invest Ophthalmol Vis Sci 1968:7:127–134.

Ken K. Nischal
Children's Hospital of Pittsburgh, Children's Hospital Drive
45th & Penn Avenue, CHP Faculty Pavilion, Suite 5000
Pittsburgh, PA 15201 (USA)
nischalkk@upmc.edu

Published online: February 16, 2021

Integrated Intraoperative Ocular Coherence Tomography for Pediatric Ocular Surgery. Dev Ophthalmol. Basel, Karger, 2021, vol 61, pp 45–51 (DOI: 10.1159/000511815)

Use of Integrated Intraoperative Ocular Coherence Tomography in Pediatric Cataract Surgery: Thinking outside the Box

Jamie L. Odden[a, b] Amani A. Davis[c] Tarek A. Shazly[b] Ken K. Nischal[a–c]

[a]UPMC Eye Center, Pittsburgh, PA, USA; [b]Department of Ophthalmology, UPMC Children's Hospital of Pittsburgh, Pittsburgh, PA, USA; [c]University of Pittsburgh School of Medicine, Pittsburgh, PA, USA

Abstract

The advent of integrated intraoperative optical coherence tomography (i^2OCT) has opened the door for safer and more complex surgeries in the retina and cornea. However, to limit its use to just two subspecialties within ophthalmology is an opportunity lost for many other subspecialties. Here, we describe the use of i^2OCT in pediatric cataract surgery in circumstances that are not traditionally considered for i^2OCT use. The specific circumstances include: evaluation and treatment of a child following cataract extraction with lens implantation who has failed two attempts at YAG capsulotomy; lysis of post-trauma keratolenticular adhesion in an opaque cornea; surgical removal of secondary lens epithelial cell proliferation after pediatric cataract extraction with lens implantation, and identification of posterior capsular openings and defects. In each case the use of i^2OCT allowed the procedure to be completed safely and successfully or informed the surgeon, allowing modification of the surgical decision tree.

Scenarios

Visual axis opacification in pediatric cataract surgery is well described, especially if the posterior capsule has been left intact. Many authors have reported that leaving the posterior capsule intact under the age of 4 years results in posterior capsular opacification. Some authors recommend leaving the capsule intact once the child is old enough to have a YAG capsulotomy performed awake, which is often the case in children around the ages of 8 years and older [1]. There are reports, however, that more than one laser procedure may be needed even in those cases where posterior capsule capsulotomy using YAG laser have been conducted. We report a child who was sent for a second opinion having had 2 YAG laser capsulotomies that failed to clear the visual axis and left the lens itself pitted [2]. Using integrated intraoperative optical co-

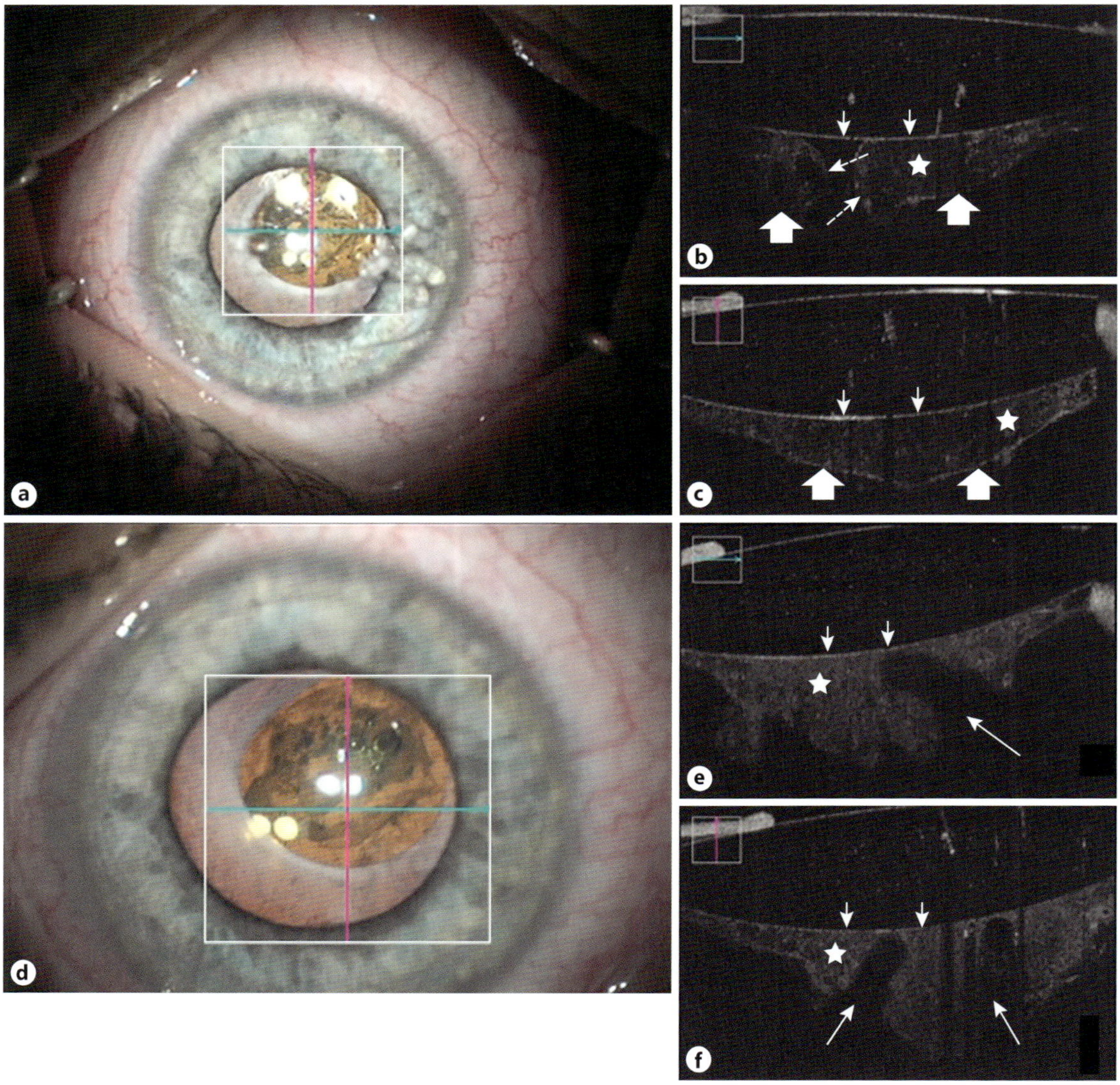

Fig. 1. An 8-year-old child who had cataract extraction with lens implantation without posterior capsulorhexis elsewhere was referred because of 2 failed YAG capsulotomies. **a** The fibrosed anterior capsule and the posterior capsular opacification. The accompanying i^2OCT (**b**, **c**) shows the posterior surface of the implant (thin short white arrows), and the posterior capsule (thick short white arrows) separated by lens epithelial cell proliferation (white star). There is one area of opening (dashed arrows), but this is isolated. **d** This finding allowed defocus of the YAG laser, after which the posterior capsule could be seen to be disrupted (**e**, **f**, thin white arrows).

herence tomography (i^2OCT), we were able to identify that the posterior capsule was sitting further away from the posterior surface of the intraocular lens (IOL) than would have been expected. As a result, we were able to offset the YAG laser focus to reflect this distance. This resulted in a successful opening of the posterior capsule. Once the posterior capsule was open

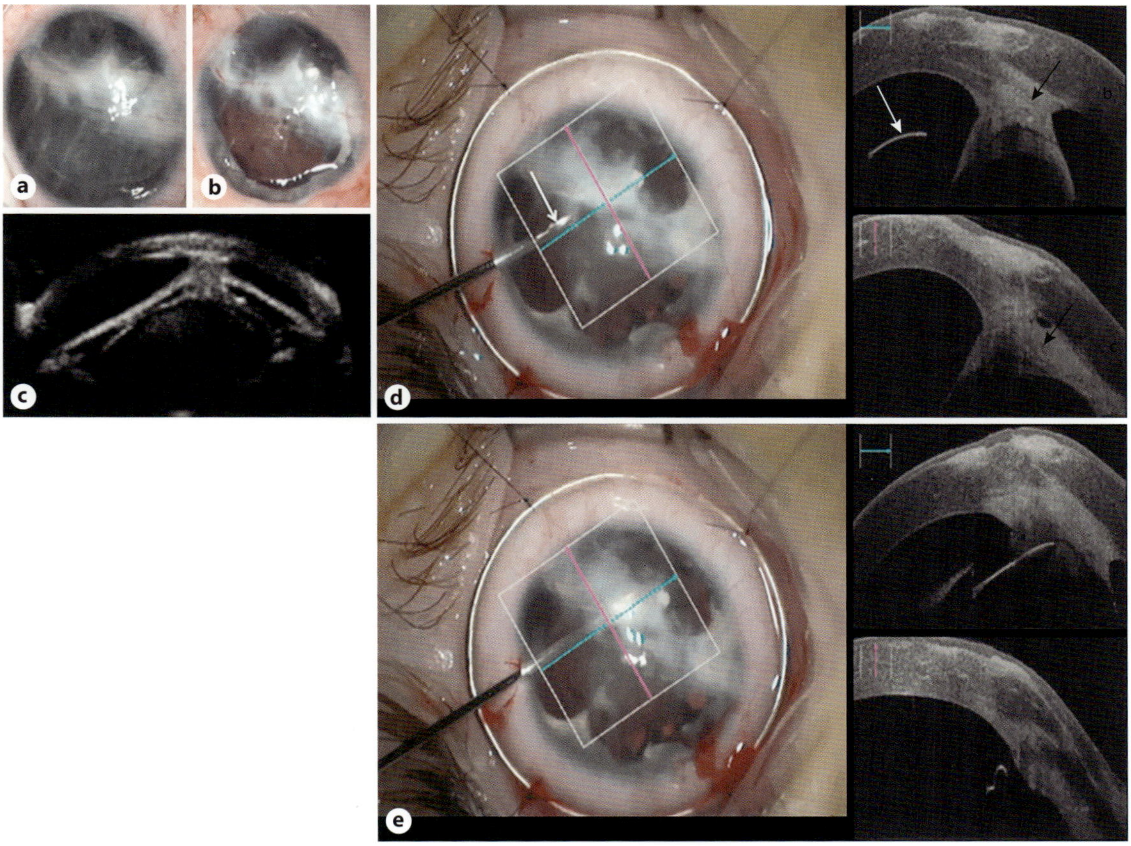

Fig. 2. A child referred after penetrating injury to the globe following primary repair. There was a vascularized corneal scar (**a**) with no visible pupil. After pupilloplasty (**b**), the lens was found to be cataractous. **c** The acquired keratolenticular adhesion can be clearly seen on high-frequency ultrasound. At operation there was no clear view of the stalk (**d**) due to the corneal scar, but using the i^{2}OCT the intraocular micro-scissors (white arrow) could be seen and did not appear to throw a shadow. **e** The stalk was cut in real time using the i^{2}OCT images.

this resulted in resorption of the lens epithelial cell proliferation resulting in gradual clearance of the visual axis (Fig. 1).

A 2-year-old male with history of left penetrating corneal injury a few months earlier presented for evaluation of left traumatic cataract. At that time, he had a left corneal scar that was large and thick, extending limbus to limbus between the upper two-thirds and the lower third of the cornea (Fig. 2a). Extending from this scar down into the supranasal part of the iris was some deep neovascularization. The cornea was otherwise clear. The lens was adherent to the back of the scarred corneal wound (Fig. 2b) on high-frequency ultrasound. The pupil was nearly completely occluded, but without iris bombe. Following pupilloplasty, the decision was made to proceed to cataract extraction, IOL implantation, and penetrating keratoplasty. i^{2}OCT provided a visual tool to tackle the keratolenticular adhesion despite an opacified cornea. The instruments used were the ordinary micro-instruments available and were not modified for use with OCT, but despite this there was no distortion dis-

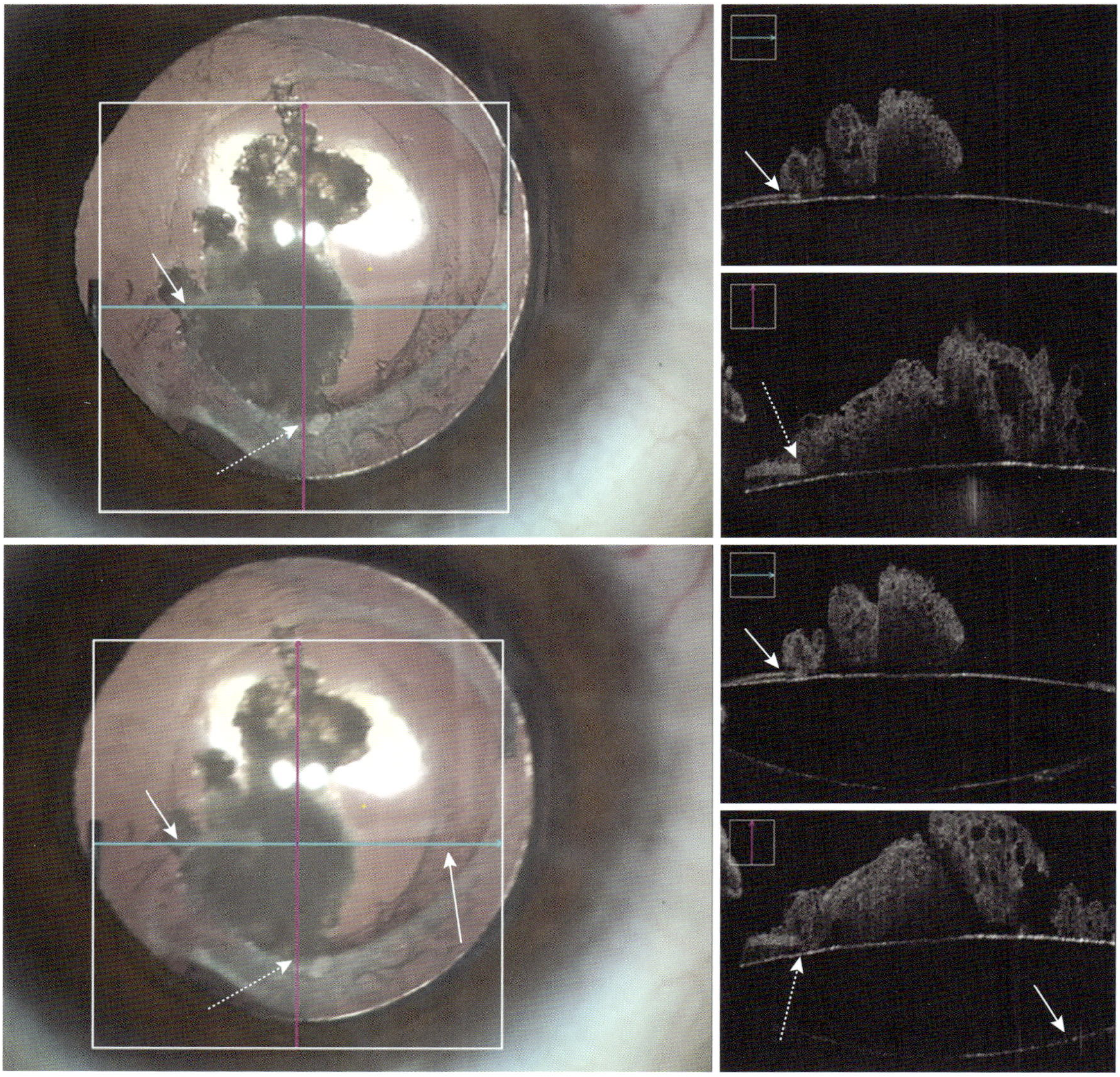

Fig. 3. Composite figure of our case at the time of removal of lens epithelial cells. External photos on the left correspond to intraoperative OCT frames on the right. The long thin white arrow shows the posterior capsule. The shorter thin white arrow depicts one point where lens epithelial cells are proliferating anterior to the lens capsule/implant interface, but note the lack of space between the capsule and the optic on the OCT. The dashed white arrow points to the area where there is expansion of new lens epithelial cells underneath the anterior capsule. The point of touch between the capsule and optic is tight. i^2OCT and the 30-G cannula allowed opening of the capsule edge from the IOL surface without tearing the capsule or causing lens tilt or decentration.

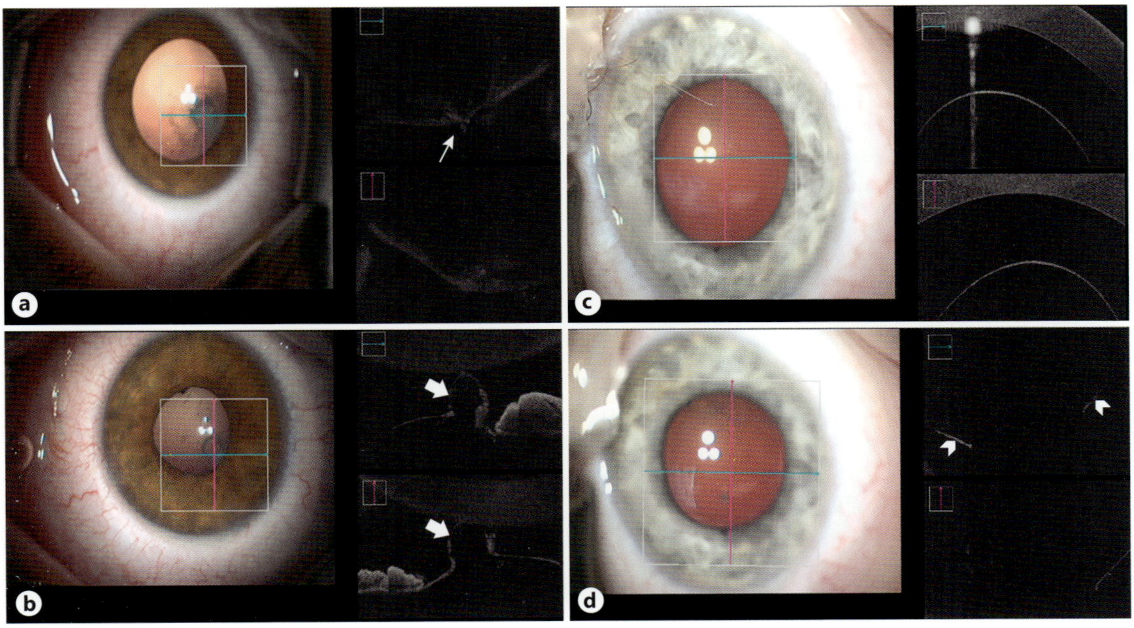

Fig. 4. The child in **a** and **b** has a posterior polar cataract which the i²OCT shows is associated with a posterior defect (white arrow). After removal of lens matter the vitreous can be seen bulging through the defect (thick white arrows). The child in **c** and **d** is 2 years old and after removal of lens matter the posterior capsule can be seen bulging forward (**c**). The novice pediatric cataract surgeon, when shown this image, will be more careful when entering the anterior chamber after lens aspiration. In **d**, a posterior capsulorhexis has been performed and the bag inflated with viscoelastic. This image shows that the elasticity of the child's capsule means that if an intraocular implant is rotated too vigorously, the leading haptic is likely to flip into the posterior segment. This is because the leaves of the posterior capsule after posterior capsulorhexis bow backwards (chevrons) when the bag is inflated with viscoelastic.

tal to the instrument outline that hindered the surgical maneuver. Separation of the acquired stalk allowed the host tissue to be trephined, followed by cataract extraction, primary lens implantation, and then donor placement and suturing. Without the i²OCT, the likely outcome would have been corneal graft with lensectomy without implantation of an IOL. The outcomes of corneal grafts where the child is left aphakic are less favorable.

A 2-year-old boy with a known diagnosis of Nance-Horan syndrome presented with a right dense cortical cataract. He had bilateral microcornea, a prominent forehead, and a small chin which gave him a slightly triangular face. He underwent standard pediatric cataract surgery with posterior capsulorhexis, anterior vitrectomy, and placement of a hydrophobic acrylic foldable IOL implant in the bag, with intraoperative photos showing thorough removal of the remaining lens epithelial cells. Eleven months postoperatively, the right eye was noted to have lens epithelial cell re-proliferation, mostly around the anterior surface of the IOL with significant obscuration of the visual axis, which has been previously reported [3]. He underwent surgical clearance of the visual axis a few weeks later using i²OCT. This allowed accurate location and determination of the extent of the proliferated lens epithelial cells, which were mainly anterior to the IOL implant in the right eye (Fig. 3). An anterior approach was performed where two stab incisions were made with an MVR blade at the 1 and 9 o'clock positions. Irrigation and aspiration cannulas were inserted and used to remove the material located centrally without insertion of the aspiration cannula between the anterior lens capsule and the lens implant due to the risk of capsular tear as illustrated by the narrow space between them on the anterior segment OCT. A 30-G cannula, which has a smaller outer diameter of 0.31 mm than the irrigation/aspiration, set with an outer diameter of 0.61–1 mm for bimanual and 1.5–1.65 mm for coaxial (or vitrectors at 0.5–1 mm), was then attached to the aspiration port and inserted between the IOL and anterior capsule under i^2OCT guidance and used to loosen and aspirate the proliferated material (Fig. 3 illustrates the tight space). This was repeated again with a 27-G cannula (outer diameter of 0.41 mm) and more lens material aspiration was possible, with residual lens material adherent. Having opened the potential space with small diameter cannulas, the aspiration cannula could now be safely inserted into the space to remove residual material toward the inner equator. We avoided the use of Healon, which is critical since it can act as a potential scaffold for re-proliferation of lens epithelial cells.

Finally, by way of two examples, it can be shown that i^2OCT is invaluable in informing the surgeon – especially one who is learning – of the anatomy of the posterior capsule, and how the decision tree can be modified. In the first case (Fig. 4a, b), the pre-incision i^2OCT shows a posterior nodular cataract but with clear evidence of posterior capsule defect. This persuaded the surgeon to remove all the peripheral lens matter first before removing the nucleus, thereby using the nucleus to tamponade any prolapsing vitreous. After lens removal the vitreous prolapse is easily seen. It was pushed back with heavy viscoelastic and a primary posterior rhexis was performed, as well as a vitrectomy.

In the second case (Fig. 4c, d), after anterior capsulorhexis and lens matter aspiration the posterior capsule can be seen bulging forward. The novice surgeon may not be aware of how much it does bulge forward in children, and so may inadvertently penetrate this when entering the eye with an instrument. Inflation of the anterior chamber with viscoelastic avoids this scenario. After performing a posterior capsulorhexis and inflating the bag with viscoelastic in children under the age of 8 years, the elasticity of the capsule means that the posterior capsule leaves the bow posteriorly (Fig. 4d). If the surgeon is not aware of this then there is a chance that vigorous rotation of the intraocular implant may result in the leading haptic flipping into the posterior segment [3].

In conclusion, i^2OCT can be used in many ways not only to attempt complex surgery, but also to inform the surgeon so that he/she may modify their surgical decision tree to get the best outcome for the child. The surgeon can adapt to it slowly, utilizing its maximum benefits for the patient [4].

Conflict of Interest Statement

K.K.N. has received honoraria from Carl Zeiss Meditech Inc. and is on the advisory board for Nevakar Inc.

Author Contributions

J.L.O., A.A.D., T.A.S., and K.K.N. fulfilled all of the following: (1) substantial contributions to the conception or design of the work; or the acquisition, analysis, or interpretation of data for the work; (2) drafting the work or revising it critically for important intellectual content; (3) final approval of the version to be published.

References

1 Elkin ZP, Piluek WJ, Fredrick DR: Revisiting secondary capsulotomy for posterior capsule management in pediatric cataract surgery. J AAPOS 2016;20:506–510.
2 Mamalis N, Craig MT, Price FW: Spectrum of Nd:YAG laser-induced intraocular lens damage in explanted lenses. J Cataract Refract Surg 1990;16:495–500.
3 Whitman MC, Vanderveen DK: Complications of pediatric cataract surgery. Seminars Ophthalmol 2014;29:414–420.
4 Ehlers, Justis P, et al: Integrative advances for OCT-guided ophthalmic surgery and intraoperative OCT: microscope integration, surgical instrumentation, and heads-up display surgeon feedback. PLoS One 2014; 9.8:e105224.

Ken K. Nischal
Children's Hospital of Pittsburgh, Children's Hospital Drive
45th & Penn Avenue, CHP Faculty Pavilion, Suite 5000
Pittsburgh, PA 15201 (USA)
nischalkk@upmc.edu

Author Index

Subject Index